Ten Commandments of Lifting Weights:

Recommendations to the Devout Bodybuilder

By: Jared Zimmerer

BEZALEL BOOKS
WATERFORD, MI

Published by Bezalel Books
Waterford, MI

Printed in the United States of America

Copyright © 2012 Jared Zimmerer

LIBRARY OF CONGRESS CONTROL NUMBER: 2012932017
ISBN 978-0-9844864-9-6

This book is dedicated to the three
most important women in my life:

To My Mother,
who taught me how to love,

To My Wife,
who possesses my heart,

And, to My Queen, Mary,
whom I long to serve.

How to Use This Book:

This book is intended to be a spiritual guideline for those who plan to become physically fit or those who have already been immersed in the physical fitness realm. The rules are meant to give advice to the reader on several different topics in order to stay away from the pitfalls of the fitness world, as well as allowing men to have an avenue of spirituality through the weight room. The call for perfection of mind, body and soul is a recurring theme throughout the book. It is written to men of all ages, there are some parts that are intended more for the spiritual beginner and some that are more advanced. I have always been intrigued by the idea of a "warrior monk", a man that is as dangerous on the battle field as he is in prayer. The weight room contains monastic-type qualities that allow for spiritual renewal and reflection upon our relationship with God. I truly believe that the weight room can become a place of sanctification and these simple rules are meant to draw you closer to the heart of God and His Catholic Church, as well as try your spiritual mettle while testing yourself physically. St. Benedict wrote his Rule for his brothers in the monastery, this is intended to be somewhat of a rule for my brothers in the weight room.

Vires et Honestas

"He has shown strength with his arm."

Luke 1:51

When a six foot five inch, 265 pound Texan gives you some firm suggestions, it's probably a good idea to follow them. When you find those suggestions are also Commandments from God Himself, then all doubt has been removed, and it's time to get down to business.

I thank God that he has provided us with such a great big Texan, in the person of Jared Zimmerer, to remind us of God's will for us regarding our own human bodies. As Christians we know that our bodies are good. God created us as ensouled bodies, as miraculous blends of the material and the spiritual. It is true that our material bodies will corrupt and decompose after our four-score years or so on earth, and that our immaterial souls will live forever — God willing — in blissful union with Him. But even then, it won't just be our souls joining God, for we will don glorified bodies, as Jesus Christ, God-made-flesh, did after His resurrection. Then, as now, we will worship and glorify God through the means of the bodies he gives us. So shouldn't we show Him some appreciation for them?

Jared's *Ten Commandments of Lifting Weights* is a most welcome addition to a small, but burgeoning field of a Catholic literature that attempts to inform and inspire us to be the best possible stewards of our God-given bodies. Robert Feeney's work, particularly his *A Catholic Perspective: Physical Exercise and Sports* opened my eyes to the blessings the Church has placed upon athleticism and the proper care of the human body, from the days of St. Clement of Alexandria (c. 150 – 215 AD) to the days of our modern popes. Indeed, as Pope Pius XII has declared, "the human body is in its own right, God's masterpiece in the order of visible creation."

Perhaps the classical idea of "a healthy mind in a healthy body," will conjure up thoughts of muscular ancient Greeks and Romans. Likewise, the modern notions of "holistic health" and "mind/body issues" will likely call to mind yoga or other Eastern religious practices. What modern Christians may not think of, but need to know, is the unmatched profundity of the Catholic Church's own teachings on proper care of body as well as soul. Again from Pope Pius XII we hear that "in the field of physical culture, the Christian concept needs to receive nothing from the outside, but has much to offer." As Blessed John Paul II, the great theologian of the body, would emphasize decades later, when it comes to the nature of man, only the Catholic Church provides us "the fullness of truth."

Mr. Feeney's writings first brought these ideas to my attention, and the more research I did a few years back, while I writing *Fit For Eternal Life: A Christian Approach to Working Out, Eating Right, and Building the Virtues of Fitness Within Your Soul*, the more I grew amazed at the truth and profundity of those ideas. For one huge example, the way St. Thomas Aquinas addressed health and virtue in his masterful Treatise on Man within the second part of his *Summa Theologica* was a springboard to the concept of using physical fitness activities in general, and strength training in particular, to grow in health *and in virtue* at the same time.

Peggy Bowes has provided a woman's touch in her contribution to the Catholic fitness world via her book, *The Rosary Workout*. It makes perfect sense to me. Every mother wants her children to be healthy, so obviously our Blessed Mother would be pleased with our efforts to care for our bodies through regular cardiovascular exercise. Now, just add a structured approach to artfully combining praying of the rosary during these aerobic workouts and you have a combination of "beads of prayer," and "beads of sweat," that is truly hard to beat. With rosary workouts we honor God and our heavenly mother *indirectly* by tending to our bodies and *directly* through prayer *at the same time*. In this way, the demands of exercise do not draw us away from our prayer life, but provide yet another avenue to heed St. Paul's words and "pray constantly."[i]

St. Paul also wrote that our bodies are the "temples of the Holy Spirit."[ii] Peggy and I, along with our author friend, Shane Kapler, and other generous contributors,[iii] tried to further heed God's call to tend our bodily temples in *Tending the Temple: 365 Days of Spiritual and Physical Devotions*. So often our well-intention plans of incorporating regular exercise and healthy eating into our daily routines get side-tracked by life's many responsibilities. Along with inspiring stories of the perseverance of the saints, we provided "exercises," indeed, most of them recommendations for literal physical exercise. And these we provided for every day of the year. We need to pray always, and always to sensibly and reverently tend to our temples as well.

This book now in your hands takes us yet another step further into the exploration and the actualization of the holy temples God has given us in the form of our fleshly bodies. I suspect that Peggy's *Rosary Workout* has especially spoken to women, though it certainly works for the manliest of men as well! *Fit for Eternal Life* and *Tending the Temple* were meant for both sexes and for all ages, though I suspect that with my emphasis upon strength training, *"Fit"* may have a special appeal to men, though it is certainly more common to see a woman lifting weights today than it was to see a man lifting them in my own teenage years (and I thank God for that!) The powerful benefits of strength training for the muscles, for bones, and for body weight control, is undeniable now, but we need to make sure we are training *the right way and for the right reasons*.

Jared's book is right on target for both. I am certain this book will appeal most to men.

In fact this book in your hands might be said to be the place where testosterone and the Holy Spirit meet. And why not? God made us as man and woman —testosterone, estrogen, and all! This book then should be read by men, and by men who would become yet more manly in the best possible sense of the word. Women too may find it of use, most especially perhaps the mothers of teenage boys who have discovered the intoxicating world of the weight room, of "pumping iron" if you will. (Old-timers used to call it "getting bitten by the iron bug.")

For boys thus bitten, there is truly a lot of poisonous information out there. The guidance found in most modern muscle magazines can endanger a boy's body with advice that leads to overtraining, and perhaps to the abuse of supplements, steroids, or other harmful substances. And as for the soul, the inducements to train are most often pride, and judging from the ads, clearly lust too. This book will be a godsend to Catholic mothers who would seek to put good and godly advice in their son's hands. And this is advice that comes from a good and godly man who has paid his dues in the weight room, in building his own prodigious strength, and in instructing and guiding groups of other grown men and youths in the proper training of both body and soul. Jared's counsel in these pages will ensure that men and boys bitten by that iron bug shall become not mirror-gazing beachcombers, but "warrior monks of the gym!"

I can heartily endorse and recommend the book you are about to read. Jared addresses the way to lift weights to glorify God, not oneself, while incorporating thoughtful reflections on prayer, devotion to Mary, Christian masculinity, the value of pain, suffering, self-mortification, and achieving difficult goals — not to mention proper gym etiquette, and sensible, effective, efficient HIT (high intensity training) strength workouts. (HIT really works, while leaving one plenty of time for life outside of the gym.)

Though Jared's approach is most sensible and reverent, any truly manly bodybuilder or weightlifter is going to appreciate advice like how to incorporate "skull crushers"[iv] into their workouts. They will also savor advice like this (after proper cautions on training noises within crowded gyms are provided): "If you are in a home gym with some buddies, then some cave-man grunts are ok." (I heartily agree.)

Well, that's enough of the appetizer. It's time now for Jared's main course. I think you will find it most nourishing, both for the body and soul. Christ told us to love God with all our heart, and mind, and strength, and soul. So now Jared, you're up. Show us how. It's time to get pumped up — about becoming the men God wants us to be!

Kevin Vost, Psy. D

---

[i] Thessalonians 5:17
[ii] I Corinthians 6:19
[iii] Authors Cheryl Dickow, Theresa Doyle-Nelson, Lisa Mladnich, & Matt Swaim.
[iv] This simply refers to lying triceps extensions (also called French presses) in which one lies on a bend with elbows high and lowers the barbell to one's forehead. When executed with proper form no actual skull-crushing is involved!

I

Thou shalt not forget
Who gives thee strength

Be conscious of the fact that the greatest honor and the most holy destiny of the body is its being the dwelling of a soul which radiates moral purity and is sanctified by divine grace.

The Catholic Ideal: Exercise and Sports, Robert Feeney

In the book of Judges, Samson, a muscle bound fighter that God endows with unbelievable strength, reaches into the heart of strength training and the dangers that can be associated with it. Samson's abilities are unrivaled, he killed a lion with his bare hands; he also kills 1,000 Philistines with the jawbone of a donkey. He was a well-known devotee to the God of Abraham, Who blessed him with the renowned mane known to give him his Herculean strength. Cutting the story short, Samson falls in love with a woman from the Philistine tribe, the enemies of the Hebrews, who ends up betraying him by cutting off his locks, causing Samson to lose his strength. In his time of weakness, the Philistines capture Samson, tie him between two pillars inside of a temple named Dagon and curse his God and test his weakness. Repentant of his sin, Samson then asks God to give him strength one last time so that he might spite the enemies of the one, true God. God grants him this wish and Samson pulls the two pillars down, destroying the pagan temple and killing the Philistines, killing himself as well. God used Samson to punish the Philistines despite his weaknesses. Samson is an excellent example of how to correctly use the physical strength given him, as well as what can happen to us when our gaze is taken away from Our Lord.

When he united his strength and tenacity to the will of God and gave God His due justice, Samson was unstoppable. Because he fell for the beauty and love of a woman, a temptation that all men can relate to, he no longer desired to please God and united his strength with that of God's enemies, who then took that strength away. Those of us that desire to be heroes of God must know what our strength is for and how to properly use it. This book is meant to help men draw into a deeper union with God through our physical nature; I will define what real strength is and how to take full advantage of the spiritual growth that can occur in the weight room. God is the ultimate strength-Giver and body-builder, if we forget this we are doomed to follow in the footsteps of Samson. In this first chapter I am going to explain strength, more specifically the three types of strength and their divine callings, in addition to describing how lifting weights increases all three of them.

Physical strength is clearly one of the main goals of strength training. Men love to see strength in action: the World's Strongest Man competitions, football, and most any other sport can be very addictive to watch. Part of the draw of physical strength is that it can encourage and inspire young men and women to better themselves. For example, Charles Atlas, or Angelo Siciliano by birth, was born a scrawny little Italian kid that was picked on for most of his life. One day when he decided he had enough and wanted to change his physique and stature, it changed his life. At his peak Atlas was receiving so much fan mail that he needed up to 30 women to help him open and sort it, almost all of the mail from young men who were thanking him for his inspiration to become better men. Atlas was one of the first men to be able to deadlift a small car in the United States, many know his exercise endeavors but few know of his personal life. When Atlas turned 75, he was still exercising daily, 50 squats, 100 sit-ups, and 300 push-ups was a regular routine. A devout Catholic known for spending his time reading scripture, when Altas' wife passed away he sought the advice of his parish priest because Atlas considered joining a monastery; his priest told him that he was too much of an inspiration to young men and women and that living the cloistered life was ill-advised. Ending his letters, "yours in perfect manhood" it was his search for self-perfection that inspired so many people to better themselves. Physical strength has many uses and aspects but even the simple attainment of strength can draw people closer to God.

One of my favorite scenes from the movie *Les Miserables* is when Jean Valjean, a hardened criminal turned devout father and politician, saves a man from being crushed to death by a cart. Because of his long years in hard labor he has become strong as an ox and is able to help this poor victim. The townspeople are amazed at his strength and are now even more gracious that he is their mayor. Using his physical strength, Valjean was able to save a human life and receive grace for doing so. This is an excellent example of how physical strength can be used for the betterment of mankind: most people do not have an opportunity to use their strength in such a heroic fashion, but all of us are called to be in a state of readiness. It takes physical strength to build a home for the homeless, or to take food to the hungry. It took physical strength for Jesus to carry the cross to the top of the hill. It took physical strength for the apostles to walk from Greece to Rome and back again.

Men were meant for hunting, farming, and hard labor, and these all attribute to physical strength. Women were meant to be able to physically withstand childbirth which requires more strength than most men have. Our time in the weight room would be irrational if we did not desire to grow in strength, agility or size. With a logical routine in use, gains should be pretty regular, even if they are on a small scale. Your body, under specific conditions, will adapt to the demands that are required, at least until your genetic potential is reached. As most of us are not blessed with the genetics of Hercules, there is a requirement of intensity in our workouts to increase beyond our means. Mike Mentzer put it this way in his book, *High Intensity Training*, "As long as our activity remains within normal limits, our muscular size/strength levels will remain essentially unchanged … In order to trigger the regulatory system into another growth cycle-growth that transcends normal adult levels of size and strength the level of our activity must be raised above normal." In other words, if you want to get strong your muscles need to be tested to their limits on a regular basis. If you are not experiencing any type of gains from consistent exercise routines, you should take a second look at the type of exercise you are performing. Whether it be muscular endurance, flexibility, or down-right strength; progression should be your goal.

The original definition of insanity: doing the same thing over and over again expecting different results. I remember when I first started lifting that the gains were very regular in size and strength but when I hit a plateau I didn't know what to do because almost all of the muscle magazines have the same high-volume, low-intensity routines to use. Then I picked up a copy of Dr. Vost's book, *Fit for Eternal Life*, in which he explains what High-Intensity Training is, and from there I started reading up on all of the rational and scientific research done by Arthur Jones, Mike Mentzer, Dorian Yates, Clarence Bass and began ignoring the Schwarzenegger worshipping culture; since then, my gains have been regular again. I highly recommend doing your homework when it comes to strength training, without the knowledge of correct and useful exercise you might fulfill that definition of insanity.

The second type of strength I would like to dive into is mental strength. We do not want to become the meatheads that the fitness world already has plenty of. In *The Intellectual Life* by the French Dominican A.G. Sertillanges, he writes, "Truth visits those who love her, who surrender to her, and this love cannot be without virtue." Since our goal is perfection, our minds must have goals and curiosities in order to grow stronger. We must learn the virtue of studiousness with the aim of growing in knowledge of our Lord and the world around us. It is sad that most people waste their time with magazines full of advertisements and pictures rather than focusing on finding a philosophy of life. God has given us the faculties to be able to grow in knowledge, the knowledge of love, wisdom and a deeper appreciation of a Creator who cares about each and every one of us. CCC #35 reads: "Man's faculties make him capable of coming to a knowledge of the existence of a personal God". Our mind is a gift; it allows us to ground ourselves in truth and to know right from wrong in order to become leaders and virtuous citizens. Our minds can stalemate if we refuse to reach beyond our comfortable little worlds of monotonous entertainment and never strive to develop our thinking abilities. The mind needs to crave for the knowledge of the unknown, because that craving will lead us to a closer understanding, and therefore love, of our Creator, and a solid exercise program will aid in the growth. "It is exercise alone that supports the spirits, and keeps the mind in vigor" (Marcus Cicero).

> **CCC# 33: The human person: with his openness to truth and beauty, his sense of moral goodness, his freedom and the voice of his conscience, with his longings for the infinite and for happiness, man questions himself about God's existence.**

Strength training and exercise give the body more energy and ability to concentrate on more important matters in life. Have you ever noticed how hard it is to think about anything after a grueling workout? Your mind is clear, the stress of the week dissipates and all seems to be right in the world. The amount of mental fortitude spent during a hard lifting session is second to none, the ability to tell yourself that despite the pain felt you will continue, allows your mind to focus and determine that the hard work will be completed. Mike Mentzer, known as the bodybuilding philosopher, devoted much of his time to reading philosophy and literature that he claimed spilled over into the gym. We should spend our time in prayer and spiritual reading and allow what we read to come with us into our workouts. Mentzer stated that in order "to be stimulated to break through mental barriers, and to perform at consistently higher levels, some unusual stimulus must fill you with emotional excitement or some idea of necessity must induce you to make the extra effort of will." That unusual stimulus that Mentzer mentions, for us who are devout Christians, should be the love and the want to honor God. The same stimulus that invigorated David to take down Goliath should be what we use in order to grow in our mental strength.

Ten Commandments of Lifting Weights

Your mind is a very powerful moving force in your life; an over-stressed mind can cause the aging process to quicken or sickness to evolve. It is also that engine behind your success in the gym and the goals you want to achieve. Through the weight room and the necessary mental calisthenics of reading literature that challenges how we think, we can not only increase the credentials of our opinions but also help ourselves to become better tools for evangelization. One of the most difficult books I have ever read was the philosophical work by Karol Wojtyla, better known as Blessed John Paul II's *Love and Responsibilty*. I have never been so challenged mentally, but by the end of the book my thoughts about who I was as a human being and weightlifter have never been the same. It is said that competition drives men to do amazing things; we should compete against our own desires of ease and comfort to become the "supermen" we are all called to be. Holiness can be learned through study because the more you fill your mind with deeper contemplations, the closer you come to the heart of your being, Jesus Christ Himself.

Spiritual strength, the central force of all three strengths, is required to grow as a spiritual warrior. Without a strong soul a strong body is useless. The union between our souls and our bodies is so intimate that we can participate in the spiritual through the physical and vice versa. "The unity of soul and body is so profound that one has to consider the soul to be the form of the body" (CCC# 365). As we grow stronger, we will come upon new roadblocks on our journey, each one requiring a renewed sense of vigor, coincides

> **"The body is for the soul as the tool is for the craftsman."**
> **—Thomas Aquinas**

with our spiritual lives. Constantly bombarded by new ways to sin, we must learn in some way how to overcome these temptations; in other words we must enlarge our spiritual muscles to take on the weight of the world as it continually gets heavier and heavier. Our bodies are meant to be in use of our souls, therefore an inadequate soul keeps the body from reaching its full potential.

Fulton Sheen once said that "A dead fish can still go along with the current; it takes a fish with life to go against it." Spiritual strength is our motivating energy to stand up for what is right and to live a life of virtue and fulfillment. I remember my senior year of college at a state university; I decided to keep the ashes on my forehead all day for Ash Wednesday. I remember the feeling I received for standing up for my faith and to not be afraid to let the world know that I was Catholic; it is indescribable. (I also had the opportunity to discuss Ash Wednesday and the Faith with an atheist, very enjoyable.) Pushing through the roadblocks along the way in the gym can and should overlap into our ability to stand up for our faith.

In Aquinas' *Shorter Summa #128* he writes that, "A modification in the sensitive appetite tends to bring about a change in the will (which is a rational appetite)." In other words as we control the appetite of our lower nature (our emotions and desires) by the influence of our higher nature (the image and likeness of God) we can cause an immediate change in our own wills, or spiritual strength.

Using one of the many stories of the Greek gods, most people do not attribute Hercules' strength to that of his humanity, being that he was half god his power came from his divine nature. People attribute his strength to the spiritual side of his life. Why do we, who are all made in the image and likeness of God, take away from the supremacy of a powerful soul? It was his magnanimity, or strength of soul, that made Hercules great, we too have a divine nature and we must work to grow in our strength of soul. Edward Sri, in an article for *Lay Witness Magazine*, put it this way, "The magnanimous person pursues greatness in proportion to his ability. He humbly takes stock of all the gifts that God has given him and seeks to use them as best he can. As Aquinas explains: Magnanimity makes a man deem himself worthy of great things in consideration of the gifts he holds from God." Greatness of soul is increased through an honest humbling of our own egos, to become heroic or legendary; humility is the first disposition we must obtain, allowing our Divine nature to have control over our lower nature leads to humility worthy of true strength training.

> **"The Iron is the best antidepressant I have ever found. There is no better way to fight weakness than with strength. Once the mind and body have been awakened to their true potential, it's impossible to turn back." (Henry Rollins, Former Bodybuilding Champion)**

In chapter 3 of Lorenzo Scupoli's *Spiritual Combat* he states, "in ourselves, we are nothing, and that dangerous misfortunes continually threaten us, reason itself suggests distrust of our own strength. But if we are fully convinced of our weakness, we shall gain, through the assistance of God, very great victories over our enemies." If we rely completely upon our own devices we will be doomed to fail in our fitness goals. People may ask, then what about all of these athletes and bodybuilders that are basically agnostic? In answering this question I propose that the athletes who do not desire fulfilling the will of God through their talents and abilities are digging their own graves. Denying God what is already His is a sure-fire way to deny yourself what is already yours, that being a place in heaven.

The *Catechism of the Catholic Church #396* says, "God created man in his image and established him in his friendship. A spiritual creature, man can live this friendship only in free submission to God" Our Creator gave us the dexterity and faculties to do wonderful things with our created bodies. In so doing He blessed us with the freedom to do extraordinary deeds, or the freedom to use them to do terrible deeds. The outcome of which we choose will be decided on the level of your dependence on God. Lest we forget that we are dependent on our Lord for the very air we breathe we are short-changing ourselves in the growth of strength and robustness. Complete self-mastery, which should be the goal of anyone entering the weight room, relies on the unifying of our minds, bodies, and most especially our souls towards the love of God. All three of these faculties have their own strengths and individually can increase through a life of strength training.

Aside from lifting weights, as Catholics, I would be remiss to neglect the divine strength contained in the Holy Eucharist. I think Blessed Pier Giorgio, another saintly bodybuilder, said it best, "I urge you with all the strength of my soul to approach the Eucharistic Table as often as possible. Feed on this Bread of the Angels from which you will draw the strength to fight inner struggles, the struggles against passions and against all adversities, because Jesus Christ has promised to those who feed themselves with the Most Holy Eucharist, eternal life and the necessary grace to obtain it." (July 1923) For about 3 years now I have been attending Mass at least 2–3 times during the week, not counting Sunday obligation. In that time I have noticed a substantial amount of growth in my fight against temptation. When we take Communion we must realize that we are literally uniting ourselves with God! Jesus Christ's body, blood, soul and divinity are intermingled into our weak and desperate humanity. The fitness world offers amazing amounts of supplements in

> **The Catechism of the Catholic Church says that God showed His love to us "By embracing in His human heart the Father's love for men, Jesus "loved them to the end...In suffering and death His humanity became the free and perfect instrument of His divine love which desires the salvation of men. Indeed, out of love for His Father and for men, whom the Father wants to save, Jesus freely accepted His passion and death."**
> **(CCC #609)**

order to grow in muscularity; this sacrament is what the Church offers to grow in magnanimity. If you want true power, power over your own self, then the Eucharistic table is the hotbed of grace. The need for us to have a soul as beautiful and well-built as our bodies can be fulfilled in the devout reception of our Lord.

When talking about strength and the Eucharist it is quite impossible not to talk about love, God is identical with both love and strength, and therefore love and strength are one in the same. In John Paul II's *Theology of the Body* it says, "The truth and the strength of love show themselves in the ability to place oneself between the forces of good and of evil that fight within man and around him, because love is confident in the victory of good and is ready to do everything in order that good may conquer" (*TOB* 115:2). Love is that all-encompassing emotion that can drive a man to take the hill for love of country or can drive him mad for the love of a woman. There is no greater virtue than love and for that reason strength residing in love is invulnerable. Being that love can be an emotion or a Being our strength owes allegiance to it simply because it is the dominant power. The philosopher Seneca stated that, 'Love in its essence is spiritual fire', our hearts, a muscle in its own right, can burn with this spiritual fire to grow in love with our God and our neighbors.

A man is nothing without his heart (love) behind his strength. St. Thomas Aquinas, in his Summa Theologica, explains it this way, *a man's strength whether spiritual or corporal depends on the heart.* In order to be a leader and a future saint, our hearts must be the driving force behind our strengths. Our hearts must be behind all three strengths in order to grow. Strength has many different forms and possibilities. Focusing on only one type of strength can delude us to think that our possibilities have limits. "I can do *all* things through Christ who strengthens me" (Philippians 4:13). We are the salt of the Earth and therefore all of our strengths and different talents help make up what is beautiful in His creation.

"Thou shalt love the Lord thy God with thy whole heart, and with thy whole soul, and with thy whole strength" (Deuteronomy 6:5).

There are many places to find strength, an example from my own life was when my children were born, I am dumbfounded by the strength and courage that my wife displays during childbirth. I literally got weak at the knees, so much so that the nurses made me sit down. To this day I still believe that my body could not handle being in front of pure God-given, feminine strength. This amazing gift of strength is all around us and we amaze at its power even though we do not recognize it at times. Jesus has shown us what true strength of body and the will can achieve. One of the few hopes that the people of God should be able to depend upon is the strength of the men around them.

In the Old Testament while the people of Israel were carrying the Ark of the Covenant, God gave very specific orders to be carried out while carrying this holy object. The relationship between God and His creatures requires a certain amount of duty towards each other. Pope John Paul II's, Love and Responsibility, explains the reciprocal relationship between ourselves and our Creator, "When we speak of justice towards God we are saying that He too is a personal being, with who man must have some sort of relationship. Obviously this position presupposes knowledge and understanding of the rights of God on the one hand and the duties of man on the other." Endowed with strength we must nourish and use the qualities given us by our Creator as justice demands. Since our bodies are gifts from God we must have dignity and respect for it, we should keep our temples in good shape, not for glory for ourselves but for God and God alone. In John Paul II's *Theology of the Body*, he really helps us understand what our bodies are for and the connection between our physical states and our spiritual states. Our bodies can either be a great gift given by God or it can be our ultimate downfall. The most common of the mortal sins committed today are through our own physical bodies, so by giving glory to God while we discipline our bodies, I truly believe that we can generate the Holy Spirit within ourselves.

Suggested Prayer

My God, my King and my Lord, I give all of the strength that you have blessed me with to You and the mission to save souls. If I were to ever deny You anything that makes me who I am as a child of God, please take it from me in order that I realize where my strength belongs, to You and You alone. Make me the spiritual warrior that all of us are destined to be. If it be in Your most holy will allow me to lead in anyway that I can. Never let me forget where true strength comes from.

Amen

II

Thou shalt always give the glory of muscularity to God

'The unity of the human person also means that his actions are not isolated events but form part of a continuum which makes him the sort of person he is. They are part of his biography. They are all moral acts, if done consciously and freely, in the sense that they lead him nearer to his last end and supreme good, or further away from it. Insofar as they lead to it, they enhance his human dignity. Moral life for man consists then, in the right ordering of all his activities to a unified end.'

– Peter E. Bristow The Moral Dignity of Man

In John Paul II's *Theology of the Body* it discusses how he felt compelled to take the loin cloths off of the pictures in the Sistine chapel, of which prudish clerics painted on so many years ago. When asked what the difference is between those glorious pictures of Michelangelo and Hugh Hefner's idea of the human body are, he replied, "One must look at the intention of the artist." Hugh Hefner's intent is to incite lust in a man and to make money off of the sins of others. Michelangelo on the other hand wanted to show men and women in the superb state that God originally intended for us to see each other. No shame of the differences between a man and a woman, God made us the way we are therefore our bodies are beautiful. If a person that exercises and lives a healthy lifestyle with the intent to make others fear them or to cause the other sex to lust after them, this mode of thinking is not what God intended at all. Whereas if a man hits the weights, diets and lives the lifestyle of a healthy, prudent adult for the glory of a gift provided by a loving Creator, then the intent is not to bring glory upon himself but upon the majesty that is the body which God has given us. Giving God his due glory through our appearance reminds me of the words of St. Francis of Assisi, "Preach the Gospel at all times, use words when necessary." While glory of muscularity can cause vanity, something I will touch on later, disciplining of the body, the weakest part of what we are, for the glory of God, can and will bring the light and radiance of Christ to others.

The devil takes gifts meant to be good, true, and beautiful, such as health, and make them into something to incite sinfulness in us in order that we might sin more against God through His own gifts. Just as the world is now obsessed with the sexual union, something that God meant for us to have in order to partake in a small taste of the heavenly love, a very similar case has happened to men and their strength and bodies. We worship athletes and athletics at these "churches" that we call stadiums and arenas. The bodybuilders today are looked at as some herculean Greek gods rather than men. The sad part is that the strength we are seeing in these athletes is just a glimpse of what could really be achieved if we gave the glory of all of our achievements to God. Just as Pope John Paul II is calling people to the real meaning of sex and almost a sexual healing of our world, I am calling men to appreciate what God has given us from the day He created us from dust. "He made the nations of the earth for health: and there is no poison of destruction in them, nor kingdom of hell upon the earth" (Wisdom 1:14). Our bodies were given to us to worship God and in its full potential it can portray a beautiful gift from heaven. Blessed Pier Giorgio Frassati used to take students on climbs up the mountains to show them what it is like to strive to reach the heavens, the pure and divine. In this same way I would like to summon you to the striving for the perfection of a gift from God, each as individual and beautifully different as the buds of a rosebush but even the most beautiful rose can wither and die without proper care and sunlight.

> *"As human beings, we need the sign of the body not only to speak about the spiritual mystery of God, but to encounter it." — Christopher West, Theology of the Body Explained*

The appreciation for a beautiful body should be directed to the admiration and gratitude of the Creator of that body. Nature, for instance, is likewise something beautiful to be treasured and justly looked upon in awe, but, the appreciation for nature must go to a thanksgiving of the Creator. In a poem by St. John of the Cross he says,

Let us rejoice, O my Beloved!
Let us go forth to see ourselves in Thy beauty,
To the mountain and the hill,
Where the pure water flows

In this poem John of the Cross shows us how we can see God Himself in the beauty of the things and material that He has created. When out in nature we tend to feel more at peace and have a real sense of what beauty is. We can literally feel the presence of God. This is the same kind of appreciation we should have for our bodies and the bodies of others. Realizing that we are created in the image and likeness of God we should do all that we can to keep it in the best of health. One would not throw trash into the ocean or burn down a forest because of the respect that they have for the creation, which in retrospect is respect for the Creator. We should view our bodies as something beautiful and a gift, it is not ours to do with as we please and ruin the in the name of "freedom".

So what is proper glory? The dictionary defines it as great honor and admiration won by doing something important or valuable. Any small act that we do for the greater glory of God gives great honor and admiration, even worship, to Him, whether it is taking care of our kids, evangelizing or standing up for what is right, all glory is due to God. C.S Lewis, in his essay, The Weight of Glory, writes "Glory suggests two ideas to me, of which one seems wicked and the other ridiculous. Either glory means to me fame, or it means luminosity." He concludes that glory should be understood in the former sense, but states that one should not desire fame before men (human glory), but fame before God (divine glory). We give proper glory to our Creator by the attitude we have towards our own bodies. Christopher West, quoting JPII put it this way, "the meaning one attributes to his body determines that person's attitude in his way of, *living the body* ... how we live as bodies ... will flow from the attitude of our hearts regarding the meaning of our bodies, the meaning of our sexuality, and the meaning of life itself." In other words, if we see our own bodies as an abstract piece of meat rather than the encapsulation of an immortal soul, we degrade who we are as human beings and therefore any glory due to God is wasted.

In a book by Kevin Vost called Fit for Eternal Life he quotes Pope Pius XII, who had a gymnasium installed in the Vatican, when he says that exercise remains in proper proportion when it:

☑ Does not lead to worship of the body;

☑ Strengthens and energizes the body rather than draining it;

☑ Provides refreshment for the spirit;

☑ Does not lead to spiritual sloth or crudeness;

☑ Provides "new excitements" for study and work; and

☑ Does not disturb the peace and sanctity of the home.

So, you see a balance of mind, body and soul can be achieved as long as a person keeps their priorities in check. Being that we are all made up of a mind, a soul, and a body, and true balance derives from the continual up-reach towards heaven of all three, our bodies must be on that celestial ladder just as much as our minds and souls should be. Servant of God Fulton J. Sheen once said, 'Peace is not a passive, but an active virtue.' Our bodies will never have peace unless we are *actively* pursuing the peace we crave which will only come about when we have full control of our passions and a healthy and active exercising life can help us achieve that temperance.

"For no one hates his own flesh but rather nourishes and cherishes it, even as Christ does the church, because we are members of his body" *(Ephesians 5:29).*

One of the many benefits of a healthy lifestyle is, for instance, when a person looks into a mirror and likes what they see, the person is more willing to stand up in public and let their voice be heard all because they are happier with themselves. This is very hard to achieve in our secular world today. Everywhere you look there is an even skinnier model or an even better looking guy who all says that they have a two week cure for belly fat (impossible by the way) or some other crazy scheme. Hard work and dedication are the one and only things that will work. "For wherever the perfection of anything tends, progress is always an approach towards the same thing." — Epictetus, *Discourses.* Just like your prayer and spiritual life if you don't put your 'nose to the grindstone' every single day you will fall off of your plans. The old saying, "No pain, No gain" falls right into place here, if you aren't willing to commit yourself and see the goal reached then failure is the only outcome. Now, that being said, I beyond a doubt believe that if we bring God and the saints into the gym with us our diet and exercise plans will prevail. Ever wonder why 99% of the population stays on a diet for at most two weeks? This is precisely because God is not in their minds when they are trying to achieve their goals. When their goal is to look better for themselves and not God, of course it is going to fail. God sees you turning away from him, so He being the great Father Figure, is going to keep you in line with failure.

Men naturally want the respect of their peers; this is because men are natural protectors. Their instincts will tell them who and what might be a threat to their family and loved ones, therefore they want their bodies to be in a condition of letting others know that he is the head of his family, and so predators beware. Women typically want to improve their bodies because by nature they want to be desirable. Women are meant for a receptive type of love by their heavenly design, whereas men have a love of giving. This is shown by our very bodies and more in depth in John Paul II's *Theology of the Body.* The new "culture of the body" presented by Arnold Schwarzenegger types, in which we are meant either to use others or to be used by others, is a dangerously skewed way of seeing the reasons behind men's physique. Again Christopher West states it this way,

> **The Catechism of the Catholic Church #2519 states, 'Purity of heart is the precondition of the vision of God. Even now it enables us to see according to God, to accept others as "neighbors;" it lets us perceive the human body — ours and our neighbor's — as a temple of the Holy Spirit, a manifestation of divine beauty.'**

"The more we grow in mastery of ourselves, the more we experience a proper ethos of seeing." Mr. West continues saying "we come to an ever greater awareness of the gratuitous beauty of the human body, of masculinity and femininity." The more we discipline our own bodies and minds in the proper view of a sacramental the more we will appreciate and admire the creation of man as man and woman as woman.

A man's muscles have many different purposes; we provide shelter and protection, we grow in affection with our wives and our family, we also have the ability to inspire our sons and daughters to have a certain view of masculinity. Why do you think kids love wrestling with their dads? Girls naturally want the touch of masculinity and boys want something to look up to and to test their own strengths. Muscles are our very engine to what and who we are. Our bodies are not curses that need to be put in their cages and never let out. We are made in the image and likeness of God therefore through our bodies we can give glory to God for that reason alone. We are made to look like God! (Although imperfectly) As it says in 1st Chronicles chapter 16:11 "Look to the Lord in *His strength*; seek to *serve Him constantly.*" Why take our muscles, gifts from God directly given to us to serve Him, and not help them grow to their full potential? Our muscularity has been given to us to show an outward sign that we are men.

In the *Catechism of the Catholic Church* under the title, The World was created for the glory of God, it says,

> "The glory of God is man fully alive; moreover man's life is the vision of God: if God's revelation through creation has already obtained life for all the beings that dwell on earth, how much more will the Word's (Jesus') manifestation of the Father obtain

life for those who see God." The ultimate purpose of creation is that God "who is the creator of all things may at last become "all in all", thus simultaneously assuring His own glory and our beatitude." (#294 parentheses added)

So, the glory of God comes to face when a man is fully living his life as a masculine leader and accepting his masculine role. In this passage it says that Jesus will give us true life when following the example He has given us. In Jesus' pattern He shows us how all the glory that we earn here on earth is due to the Almighty. When Jesus was in the garden of Gethsemane, sweating blood, he gave us real example of how especially at the hardest times of our lives, the mission must be completed and the glory must go to God. If Jesus wanted to keep the glory all He had to do is come off the cross and let the world worship Him, by allowing His life to be taken so that we might have eternal life, He is giving all the glory to God the father by executing God's will and not His own.

In the first commandment, "I am the Lord your God, you shall have no other gods besides me", our Lord is asking something of all of us. Of course, we are not to worship false idols (power, pleasure or possessions) but I believe He is asking

'Was it for nothing that God gave you eyes and endowed them with breath so keen and refined that it spans the distance to objects, and assumes their shape? ... So don't be ungrateful for these gifts, but at the same time don't forget that there are others superior to them ... the faculty intended to use them, to test them, and to judge their relative worth'
— Epictetus, Discourses.

for so much more here. When we give God the due glory of every one of our movements, actions, even every beat of our hearts, we give Him the pride to know that we worship Him and Him alone. Many of the saints, St. Therese of Liseux for instance, have shown us how to give every single moment we have to God and to constantly strive to be alongside Him, walk with Him, in everything we do. Men are physical beings, born to have muscle and to use those muscles for the purpose God gives us. Our muscles are blessings, and when we start seeing them that way and giving the glory of them to God and God alone we will see a steady decline in obesity, depression and despair. We will see an increase in devoted prayer lives and fathers that are more than willing to sacrifice everything that they have for their families and the entire communion of saints.

One thing I have always heard is that the choirs of angels are only envious of human beings for one reason: The Holy Eucharist. Our bodies are the sacramental vessels in which the Body, Blood, Soul and Divinity of God-made-man enters into our souls. You would not want the Church you enter for the Sacrifice of the Mass to be filthy or in need of repair, parishioners pay large amounts of money to keep the parish looking at its best. In the same way, keeping our bodies pure and undefiled through healthy eating habits and an exercise regimen is like helping your Creator tie the ribbon around the gift He gives you. "For this is the Will of God, Your sanctification; that you abstain from immorality; that each one of you know how to control his own body in holiness and honor" (1 Thessalonians 4:3–4).

Suggested Prayer

My Lord, my God, and my King I thank you for the muscles you have blessed me with as a man. May I use them in your will and give all the glory that they bring to You and You alone. Jesus show me what it took for you to carry that cross so far for so long. May I, like Simon of Cyrene, help you with the horrible burden I have given you through my sins. I want to be a warrior at the top of my potential, teach me and show me how.

Amen

III

Thou shalt use this time for self-realization and mortification

"The world, looking on, sees that devout persons fast, watch and pray, endure injury patiently, minister to the sick and poor, restrain their temper, check and subdue their passions, deny themselves in all sensual indulgence, and do many other things which in themselves are hard and difficult. But the world sees nothing of that inward, heartfelt devotion which makes all these actions pleasant and easy."

–Francis De Sales

Every man is tested in their faith. The devil and his minions can speak into our ears and lead us down roads we never dreamed of stepping foot on. If a man has confidence in himself and in God he tends to be able to handle more opposition. This can be seen through everyday events. For instance, if a man and his family happened to be approached by a mugger or robber which man is going to react quickly and decisively, the man that has no confidence in his own strength or the man that has been working on his body and knows his strengths and that he can handle this other man? I don't know about you but I would much rather be the man that is confident and able to protect his family and fulfill his masculine duty. Now in the spiritual sense, think of it in the same way. If a temptation to sin arises which man is going to be able to overcome? Obviously it is the man that knows his own strengths and weaknesses. When an attack comes, this man will be prepared because he admits to his weakness therefore has already taken the first step to overcoming it. So even if there is a fall he will be able to get back up sooner than if he denied it was a problem at all.

When a man is lifting weights he can feel exactly where his strengths and weaknesses reside. This leads to self-realization, or realizing who we are as men.

(Now, when I talk about self-realization, I am not talking about the pagan Hindu practice! Do not think that is where I am headed with this. Their definition has nothing to do with God.) A man likes to know exactly what he is capable of, most of the time for a deeper meaning. For example, most men would like to know how to build a fire, hunt, or be able to make a shelter out of nothing but what the woods offers to them. This isn't some macho man thing to know, it's specifically because it is in their nature to want to know. Men are born to be providers and protectors of their families. Most men will never be put in a situation where these skills would be needed these days but the want will always be there. Just as in the weight room a man wants to know what he is capable of so that deep down inside he comes to know himself better than he did before. Most people these days are living lives that don't really feel define who they are. We fall into this trap of a safety net and leave all of our wants and dreams aside because it isn't practical. But I think the problem goes even deeper than that. Most of us don't even know who we really are.

We let our jobs, money, stature, and toys define who we are while the screaming "real me" inside of us is just waiting to have a chance to show you who you are. When a person is lifting weights all the money, stature, etc. have nothing to do with what is going on. It is the real you staring yourself in the face and asking you, "are you willing and able to go to war with me?" This is the same question that our heavenly Father asks us every day, so in turn when a person comes to terms and is able to accept who and what they are, they will be much more willing to go into battle with the saints and angels. Men who hunt and fish on a regular basis almost always are more confident and able to make decisions for their families. Most people have realized that the men that come out of the military are all very

*"**Muscle shape, leanness, and a strong, healthy system are the early motivators, worthy and always before us. However, if you expect that the benefits of iron are limited to those goals only, then you are in for a grand surprise. Look for, better yet hunt for, and gather the riches along the way that develop solidness, depth and width to the character and mind. Each and every workout provides reward, encouragement and good cheer. The gym experience never fails; the lifting, the straining, the winning and the losing make you stronger ... Every workout is an uncovering of fortitude, the further excavation of patience and persistence and a prosperous mining of discipline and humility."*
Dave Draper, Brother Iron Sister Steel*

confident and very relaxed in tense situations. This is because they have put themselves to the test, and have passed; therefore they have accepted who they are. A man learns a lot about himself when he puts his life and strength on the line.

Besides the physicality of working out or labor, how else might we come to know ourselves better? When we are searching for whom and what we truly are at our deepest core, the same conclusion will rise up in every man, that core is Jesus Christ Himself. So, in other words, the real question that most men should be asking themselves is can I find out how to bring the core of my being, Jesus, to head? In the encyclical *Gaudium et Spes*, it says, "Man can fully discover his true self only in a sincere giving of himself." In Carl Anderson's book, *A Civilization of Love*, he describes this passage as follows: "This implies that something in the act of self-giving reveals or causes us to realize our true nature. More important it is a promise- self-giving is not simply the act of looking for self but an act of the discovery of self." As I said before what we are all really looking for is the face of Jesus, because this is what is inside of us all. So when Jesus said, "whatever you do to the least of my people that you do unto me", I think what He was really saying is, "find yourselves in others through me." Only there can we find happiness and joy, the real face of Jesus Christ. Through the emptying of oneself we really find what we are made of. Just as when a man goes to war he finds out if he is willing to take that hill or sit back and let others fight, we find our true nature in the helping of the helpless by seeing Jesus in them.

When we give ourselves completely to someone else we realize what we are meant for in this world, love. Just as when a man and woman give themselves to each other through the marital act, new life is given, revealing both the man and the woman in the child, not only physically through the looks of the child but the mannerisms and abilities of the child portray the inner being of the parents. A man can really see what he is made of through his own children. Most men will say to others that their sons or daughters are made of everything that is good in them. In the same way when we help the helpless we can give them everything that is good in us (Jesus) in order to improve that person's life in the name of Jesus Christ. Our triune God has always and will always know Himself completely. Therefore, when He made us in His image and likeness, He allowed us to reveal who He is through our lives. So when we help others through self-less giving we are revealing not only to ourselves but to everyone around us that God, in the person Jesus Christ, is who we really are at the very core of our being and who we should all strive to emulate.

Jesus' death on the cross is the ultimate example of self-giving and selfless love. When it came to be Jesus' time to die on the cross He was well aware of who and what He was in the eyes of God. His entire life was given to others. Growing up

He gave Himself to His earthly parents. God Himself, had such a spirit of self-giving that He was willing to humble Himself down to the role of a carpenter's son and live in the shadows for 30 years. This is showing us that when we humble ourselves and give our lives over to something greater we can find out who we are as men and women. By the time He was ready for His mission Jesus had to know who He was at His core in order to let the mission be successful. His entire mission was based around self-giving, He never once put His own life before any one of ours. If we are to follow Jesus' footsteps and find Jesus in ourselves we must live in the same manner. Examples like Mother Teresa have given us inspiration to live in a state of self-donation to all, especially the poor, the young, and the helpless. We don't ask ourselves whether or not the person is worthy of our love. Why is this? It isn't by our own merit; I can guarantee everyone of that fact. But it is because in the eyes of the suffering and the lowly we see the light of something greater inside of them, something that we all want for ourselves. That light, that deep happiness is Jesus Christ living through

"As we advance in the spiritual life and in the practice of systematic self-examination we are often surprised by the discovery of vast unknown tracts of the inner life of the soul"
Basil William Maturin, Self-knowledge and Self-Discipline

His people. When we are helping others through the virtue of charity we see and feel something inside of us that makes us feel at peace, a peace that only faith and service in Jesus Christ can bring. We also feel a peace of soul that cannot be replaced by anything else in our lives. We truly feel serenity within ourselves and almost feel more 'human' when we help or when we raise our children through self-sacrifice. This level of self-giving helps us look deep inside ourselves and feel happy for who we are, which, in a world as de-humanizing as ours, this is a rarity. But that feeling of peace and serenity is what God wants for us all. We can reach that feeling through finding ourselves in the service of others.

So what other ways of self-knowledge should we strive to perfect in our daily lives? I have outlined the importance of physical self-knowledge and now I will go into the importance of spiritual self-knowledge, we are mind, body and soul after all. Concupiscence, or the natural tendency to sin, causes many a good man to fall for things that tear him away from God. Every single man in this world when diving into a spiritual self-knowledge can find mistakes and sins that he has brought upon himself, many times this can lead to despair, but true spiritual self-knowledge is more like checking off the list of "do-no-mores" that can lead a man to spiritual ruin or perfection. The soul open to grace and knowledgeable of his faults no longer dwells on his failings but realizes where they are and tries with all his might to stay away from any temptation, which is very manly. When the troubled soul falls to their knees and begs God for forgiveness, the reason they are truly sorry is because they look to the cross and see what their own faults have caused, the death of Love Itself. St. Bernard of Clairvaux, a spiritual warrior himself, thought it was of great importance to be knowledgeable of our own selves, "This is how a man becomes accursed when he is found to be ignorant of God. Or should I say ignorant of self? I must include both: the two kinds of ignorance are damnable, either is enough to incur damnation."

A self-righteous soul does not see the point in falling to their knees because they claim to be good, but, this means that they simply do not know themselves, we are all sinners. As Fulton Sheen stated in his book *Peace of Soul*, "The self-righteous man is like a white sepulcher, on the outside it is beautiful but on the inside is filled with dead men's bones." Jesus came to heal the sinners of the world, the people that knew they needed a savior. The self-righteous of the world are the one's still looking for the savior of economic problems because they see the disgust and corruption of the material world but do not see the revulsion within their own souls. We must strive to keep our souls in order or else society will reflect what is inside of all of us. To achieve this one must aim to keep their consciences clear of all self-pity and guilt through a deep examination of their own consciences.

A peace of conscience is really the only peace that we can achieve while still in this world, it is what we all long for when we cry out for the peace of God. Sheen says, "The examination of conscience brings to the surface the hidden faults of the day; it seeks to discover the weeds that are choking the growth of God's grace and destroying peace of soul." When we look to our own lives and see the wretchedness that we can achieve, our own souls and wills will be begging us to turn to Jesus for forgiveness and through this forgiveness we will be able to learn more about ourselves, which is the forerunner to self-perfection. By keeping a commitment of examining our own souls in the morning or evening, I prefer in the evening, we look to the actions of the day and ask ourselves if these actions were on the winning or losing side of the spiritual battle that we are all subjected to. Through the reflection of the day's events we can learn from our own mistakes and then achieve to correct them.

This is where the beauty of a good confession comes in to play. Without confession we would all be walking more or less as miserable wrecks from the guilt we carry through our sins. It is a truly masculine modality to drop to your knees and realize that there is something greater out there that demands your perfection and when this perfection is not lived we are losing battles for that higher Good, namely Jesus Christ. Going to war without the right training will lead to disaster and chaos. Confession is the bullwhip that can keep us on the straight and narrow and allow us to let Jesus take over our lives and therefore give us the strength and ability to live with honor, integrity, and a sense of who we are to be in this world as men. When sins still lurk on our souls the whole idea of a right and a wrong way to live becomes like looking through a window with the sunrise on the outside but the shades are down. Without this sense of right and wrong, a real sense of duty, we could never know our real selves instead we lean into this superficial way of living and consider this 'life' our own. Fulton Sheen quotes the ancient Greeks in his book *Peace of Soul* by saying that the Greeks thought that in order to live a normal life of wisdom, of sanity, was to "Know Thyself", what better way to know ourselves than through Jesus Christ, for He is who we all are looking for when we are searching for the "real me".

Self-Mortification

Jesus calls everyone to a state of self-denial. "If any man will come after me, let him deny himself, and take up his cross, and follow me" (Matthew 16:24). We are called to deny everything that we have and are in order to keep Jesus at the top of our priorities. Self- mortification is a concrete way to practice self-denial. Jesus himself fasted for forty days in order to be ready for the mission ahead. The idea of putting ourselves through pain in order to grow as a person is such a lost concept in our society these days. It's all about pleasure and what can I get out of every situation. When we have the slightest headache the first thing we do is take aspirin to kill any pain that we possibly are experiencing. Our society has shownitself as a nation of pleasure, whether through pornography, contraception, promiscuous sex, or drugs all we think about is what kind of pleasure am I going to experience next. Throughout history the most masculine countries were the ones that have been raised in harsh times and taught that life is tough and the strong survive. This is why our country was so great for a long time. When the pioneers were founding this country they went through some of the hardest times known to man. Harsh weather, dangerous natives, and killer animals never seen before by these brave souls caused them to be tough and to push through for a greater cause. Through killing any idea of pain we have made our country weak.

Saints have perfected this idea of self-denial. St. Francis of Assisi used to jump into a rose bush, thorns and all, if he ever had a sinful thought, that bush is still growing today and no longer grows thorns. St. Anthony used to whip himself with ropes if he ever had prideful thoughts. Now, I am not saying that we need to take it to this level but we do need to realize that it is better to experience a little bit of pain now rather than ever allow ourselves to stray away from God. What are we trying to do when we allow ourselves to experience pain? What we are trying to do is reach a level of self-discipline in order that we can keep our eyes on the prize which is fulfilling God's will. In the Gospels of Matthew and Mark they both say, "The spirit is willing but the flesh is weak," so by strengthening our bodies and wills, through self-denial, we can cause ourselves to be an unstoppable force. By telling our bodies no on a regular basis it becomes much easier to tell our bodies no when confronted with sinful temptations. It's the same reason a parent tells a child to brush his teeth or not to eat so many sweets all the time, in order to give them disciplines that will stay with them through their lives and help them to live happier and healthier. I truly believe this is why Jesus fasted for forty days so the He could control His body; He was 100% man after all, so that when His time came

> *The catechism says, "The way of perfection passes by way of the Cross. There is no holiness without renunciation and spiritual battle. Spiritual progress entails the ascesis and mortification that gradually lead to living in the peace and joy of the Beatitudes" (#2015)*

to go through the torture and death, He would be ready and willing and never surrender and give in to the temptation to give up. Obviously He was a little worried about the road ahead or else He wouldn't have had the agony in the garden. Jesus is constantly reminding us that it is not the proud that make it to heaven but the lowly will be exalted. When we fast and deny ourselves of certain necessities we also realize how small and dependent our bodies truly are. This is the same reason we have lent. We realize that without certain things we cannot survive, this is the similar with the soul, without God our soul would not survive.

Pleasure and pain are always related to each other, you cannot have one without the other. For example, the pain of childbirth is always followed by the much more powerful pleasure of the new child that follows. Another example is the pain of being a parent when one must scold their child so that they will have the pleasure of seeing that child grow into a responsible adult. Just as the pleasure of a heavenly afterlife was and is only reachable through sharing in the pain of the crucifixion with Jesus. There are two different types of self-mortification, the self inflicted mortification and the kind that comes our way that is out of our hands. The latter is things such as weather, people's attitudes, insults, defeat in an argument etc. In Cardinal Francis Arinze's book *Alone with God* he says, "if anyone bears these unpleasant situations with patience and love of God and with total self control and undisturbed joy, that person is on the road to sanctity," a road we should all strive to be on.

The first type of mortification, the self inflicted kind, are freely chosen acts that we deliberately allow ourselves to endure, fasting for instance. One way that men can really mortify themselves, something that results in self discipline, is lifting weights. While lifting your muscles will rip and tear and this is not a very pleasurable part of the lifting, same as the soreness that might occur the next day. But, when we teach our bodies to handle the pain of our own choices through a rigorous exercise plan, we can, I believe, learn how to deal with the pain of this world in a joyful and loving way. Jesus Himself regards mortification as a way of sanctity. Before most decisions Jesus would fast or spend an entire night in prayer and go without sleep. During His agony in the garden, before his arrest, He suffered so much anxiety that blood literally leaked out of His blessed pores. At any point in time He could have decided to stop the agonizing and crush His enemies, but knowing the will of the Father he gladly accepted the torture he was put through. His voluntary suffering redeemed us; our voluntary suffering can also clean our souls.

Redemptive suffering is the attachment of our suffering to the sufferings of Jesus on the cross. I am reminded of a quote of Mother Teresa's when she

"For example, each of us needs deliberately to mortify the appetite for food and drink according to the person's condition and good advice from his spiritual director. Failure to do this makes the person weak and liable to faults and even falls in bigger matters. Allied to the appetite for food and drink is the entire sense of feeling. The soft person seeks what is comfortable, sweet, easy, and nice-colored. He finds kneeling difficult. He does not stand erect. His movements are noisy. He sleeps longer than he should. His bed is too soft. His choice of clothes is too foppish. He is not mortified. He does not look like a disciple of Him who carried His cross up the rugged road to Mount Calvary, with a crown of thorns on His bleeding head."
Cardinal Arinze, Alone with God

was talking with one of the many sick that she attended to and the person was complaining about the terrible headaches that they were suffering from and Mother Teresa said, "Those headaches are kisses from Jesus on the cross, and the man said Mother please tell Jesus to stop kissing me." While the innocence of that statement is precious, it is really is able to portray the power of our suffering and how much Jesus loves us to embrace the cross with Him for the salvation of souls. Our sufferings are "kisses" from the cross that Jesus allows us to bear with Him so that we can come closer to his infinite love. Without suffering man would not have salvation, such is the way of justice. So, when offering up our little sufferings of the day, but also the immense ones, we are fulfilling our Catholic Christian duties in coming closer to the crucified Christ.

Now, I must speak of the fact that mortification for the wrong reasons can only end in sin. If we are to journey down the road of physical mortification for the perfection of our souls and the binding of the body and God's holy will, then we must make sure, in all circumstances that we do it out of love, love of God and love of our own God-given souls. For without love our mortification is useless. Bishop Sheen said, "Mortifications of the right sort perfect our human nature; the gardener cuts the green shoots from the root of the bush, not to kill the rose, but to make it bloom more beautifully … But they must be done from the right motive, and they must sacrifice the very things to which we wish to cling." One of the latest disorders done by teenagers these days is cutting or hurting themselves. Most of these poor souls are just crying out for attention. These mortifications are not of the right order at all, not only are they hurtful and scarring, but they take foothold in getting a sadistic pleasure out of pain. St. Anthony used to whip himself with ropes because he believed he was useless and purely sinful in the eyes of

"And if I should distribute all my goods to feed the poor, and if I should deliver my body to be burned, and have not charity, it profits me nothing"
(1 Corinthians 13:3).

God. If he were not of right mind and heart, these mortifications would have been considered masochistic, but because of his desire for holiness these simple hurts helped him in his path of holiness. A person does learn to enjoy the pain experienced in the weight room; we must make sure that we are using this pain for the right reasons.

The ultimate end that we desire is self-control and discipline in the name of love of God. Through the physicality of something as masculine as lifting weights we can not only discipline our bodies and minds but also come to the discipline of a virtuous life, I will touch on virtues in another chapter. Without the discipline of mortifications and the self-knowledge through Jesus Christ, this is not a masculine way of life. A man has a hold on his own life and does not let his instincts or urges tell him who and what he is, he allows his reason and faith in God to dictate every move that he makes, he does not allow the feelings of the moment or the fleeting desires of materialism and a secular society to even take effect into his life. Our emotions and desires can be very deceiving. A man that allows himself to be cleansed through a little bit of pain, joined together with the pain of the cross, and the growth in self-knowledge is a very dangerous man, spiritually of course, which is the goal of any man who wants to live a masculine lifestyle.

Suggested Prayer

My most Sacred Master, Jesus Christ, I give all that I am and have to You and You alone. Let my life emulate yours. I want to be firmly united to Your most sacred will, whether it calls for my life or for the denial of a few materials in this world. Help me to grow in knowledge of myself that I may come to know you better and to see You living within me. I know that I am but a wretched creature but deep within my soul, there you are living vibrantly. Help me to bring this light of your most sacred heart to the very core of my being.

Mary, Queen of the martyrs, pray for us.

IV

Thou shalt use this time to train to be a warrior for The Queen Mother, Mary, Warrior of all warriors

"In trial or difficulty I have recourse to Mother Mary, whose glance alone is enough to dissipate every fear"

— *St. Therese of Lisieux, Doctor of the Church*

In the game of chess there are many different pieces with many different characteristics and fighting abilities. There are pawns, rooks, knights, bishops, queens, and kings. If one is familiar with the game, the importances of these pieces differ. Pawns are the ones that you must sacrifice for the better of the game. Rooks, knights and bishops are very dangerous yet can be caught in traps due to their limited abilities. The king is by far the most important of all the pieces, if you lose him the game is over. The queen however is the absolute most dangerous piece on the entire board. The queen is the first piece the enemy will try and take out during the game, therefore it is the piece a player must keep safe and try to never lose her. She can move anywhere on the board and very little limits her abilities to fight off the other pieces. Such is the way of Mary.

Mary is the woman that all men crave. We see her in our wives and daughters in their innocence and majestic beauty. When men grow up thinking of the fair maiden in the tallest tower that they would be willing to fight and die for, that fair maiden that we search for is in a cave, hovering over a manger looking upon the King that will save the world. She is the woman that all women want to be when they are after a purely chaste life. When men protect their woman as a natural reaction it is the thought of what is inside of them, something man can only ponder over yet woman has perfected, innocence and purity. Mary is a model of real courage and bravery for all men and the perfect image of what woman ought to be. In the Bible she is the one that started Jesus' mission. "Do whatever he tells you" is her battle cry to all men to go to war with her. Mary is a warrior. God saved her from original sin and Jesus allowed her to suffer with Him in the salvation of the world. In Mary's *Fiat*, "Be it done unto me according to thy word", she is giving herself up to a higher cause. When the Baby is born she was the channel that God went through to save the world, what other kind of warrior is their? Fulton Sheen compares Jesus' birth as the unsheathing of a sword. That sword was raised and sharpened by the most holy woman the world has ever or will ever know.

> *"Undoubtedly, we find here an expression of the Son's particular solicitude for his Mother, whom he is leaving in such great sorrow. And yet the "testament of Christ's Cross" says more. Jesus highlights a new relationship between Mother and Son, the whole truth and reality of which he solemnly confirms. One can say that if Mary's motherhood of the human race had already been outlined, now it is clearly stated and established."*
> **— Redemptoris Mater**

The dictionary defines the word oath as a ritualistic declaration, typically based on an appeal to God or to some revered person or object, that one will speak the truth, keep a promise and remain faithful. In the beginning of the story of salvation an angel visits a humble little girl and asks her to give God a physical body. In God's infinite wisdom and justice He cannot force Himself onto anyone, pure love is not forceful. The Holy Spirit is a gentleman, he sent his wing-man the archangel Gabriel, to ask for her esteemed hand in a sharing of bringing about the Savior of the world. Gabriel then tells her, "Do not be afraid, Mary, for you have found favor with God. And behold, you will conceive in your womb and bear a son, and you shall call his name Jesus. He will be great, and will be called the Son of the Most High" (Luke 1:30–32). Every warrior in history must give an oath to fight for what is right, one to God, one to country and one to family. She had given her oath to God, as John Paul II states in Redemptoris Mater, "This fiat of Mary — let it be done unto me" — was decisive, on the human level, for the accomplishment of the divine mystery. There is a complete harmony with the words of the Son, who, according to the Letter to the Hebrews, says to the Father as he comes into the world: "Sacrifices and offering you have not desired, but a body you have prepared for me … Lo, I have come to do your will, O God" (Hebrews 10:5–7).

She gave God the oath that He may use her as He sees fit. John Paul II continues saying, "In faith she entrusted herself to God without reserve and devoted herself totally as the handmaid of the Lord to the person and work of her Son.'" Her oath to her country took place because at the time the Jewish people all knew of the prophecy of a king to come and save them. She was to be the mother of the King who brought salvation to her countrymen. She took the oath to her family (the universal family of the Catholic Church) to intercede and care for anything or anyone God put in her life. "Woman, behold your son!' Then he said to the disciple, 'Behold, your mother!' And from that hour the disciple took her to his own home" (John 19:25–27). We are Mary's family and when she said yes to God she vowed to take care of us and bring us closer to Him. Our queen is not one to take an oath lightly. At the time oaths were taken much more seriously than I think they are these days. In that day in age, to go against an oath was such a disgrace that one could barely show their faces or dishonoring a pledge could even mean death to the offender, Mary was raised never to promise something she cannot keep. And after she said yes to the angel she bowed before him and the Holy Spirit came upon her as a king would lay his sword upon a knight worthy of nobility.

The bravery that she showed that day the angel visited her could surpass even the bravery of say, a man like William Wallace, he fought for the physical world and she the spiritual. He fought for one country; she fights for generations upon generations of an entire world, and this is why, "all generations shall call her blessed," because she fights the fight that we cannot achieve ourselves. That day she knew only the joy that any mother would feel when they know there is a child, another soul, inside of the womb God uses to complete the miracle of life. But only 40 days into the life of her divine child and the cross comes hanging over her like a shadow over a lily. She was literally told that swords would pierce her heart if she was to continue in her mission to help save the world, something most people would decide to back out of. Her heart was overjoyed when she was able to raise her only son, the very Son of God, with one of the most masculine men in history, St. Joseph. She understood that it takes a real man to raise a hero and a martyr, something our world is in dire need of.

Mary is a warrior in the strictest sense of the word. Which according to the American Heritage dictionary is defined as, "One who is engaged aggressively or energetically in an activity, cause, or conflict." She gave her life to a cause and was willing and able to carry out the mission even to Calvary hill. We have another cause to belong to her and to be her warriors, that is, she is our Holy Queen Mother. The fifth glorious mystery of the Rosary is the coronation of Mary as Queen of heaven and earth. When our lady was assumed into heaven she was given a crown of stars upon her head and a throne to sit on beside her Son. In Kevin Johnson's book simply titled *Rosary* he says "A queen to the Greeks and Romans was a person who took her rank not in her own right but by virtue of the son she produced; a queen was simply a woman who produced the child of a king, or a child who became a king." As Christians we believe that Jesus is our King ruling from a throne in the form of a cross, so it would only make sense to have His immaculate mother as our sovereign queen.

Netbible.org stated that "in Daniel 5:10 the term 'malketha' ("queen,") really means the mother of the king: It stands to reason that among a people whose rulers are polygamists the mother of the new king or chief at once becomes a person of great consequence." Mary is the mother of our new King, she did not choose Him but she allowed our heavenly Father to choose her in order to have a King. Something interesting about this passage of the importance of the queen mother when it says, "among a people whose rulers are polygamists the mother of the new king or chief at once becomes a person of great consequence" in the same way we, who are all sinners, maybe not polygamists but we are

A great sign appeared in heaven: a woman clothed with the sun, and the moon under her feet, and on her head a crown of twelve stars" (Revelation 12:1).

all without a doubt sinners to the core, the mother of the new king becomes a person of great consequence, and she gives all of us a new king to wipe away the sins of old and be reborn in our new majesty with Jesus Christ.

Even during the so-called dark ages the role of the queen mother was for inspiration to the armies to fight for her. Precisely because she represented what was good and pure in the country and what the ideal glory that could come from defending her honor. A soldier knew that she was blameless and as pure as a lily and therefore the soldier was willing to fight and die for her if necessary. The queen mother was not involved in the politics of war, she was only concerned about her soldiers, their families and what was best for her country. There is a great scene in Mel Gibson's *Passion of the Christ* when Jesus is carrying the cross and He falls in a place where Mary could see Him and Mary runs to Him as any good mother would and they exchange glances of love toward each other and one could tell that Mary just wanted the suffering to stop but she knew that the mission must be completed for her beloved children, us, as unworthy as we are. And Jesus looks at His mother and says "See mother, I make all things new" and He picks up His blood-stained cross and keeps trudging one step at a time. I believe that what was being portrayed was the ability of Mary to cause a man to keep going in the name of our heavenly Father, just a glance of love gave Jesus that little bit of adrenaline to get back up and keep moving.

In St. Louis de Montfort's book *The Secret of Mary* he states that, "Mary, the Mother of the living, gives to all her children portions of the Tree of Life, which is the Cross of Jesus. But along with their crosses she also imparts the grace to carry them patiently and even cheerfully; and thus it is that the crosses which she lays upon those who belong to her are rather steeped in sweetness than filled with bitterness ... The consolation and joy which this good Mother sends after the trial encourage them exceedingly to carry still heavier and more painful crosses." This statement not only brings forth the spiritual abilities of our Lady but also the necessity of a love and devotion for her. I have heard it said that all the devil would have to do is utter the sweet name of Mary and all would be forgiven, this is so invigorating for all of us, while we may not be the devil we are all wretched sinners in need of a mother's love. In Lorenzo Scupoli's book *Spiritual Combat* he compares Mary to an empty bottle of perfume. Everyone knows by experience that the empty bottle still keeps that aroma of the sweet smelling liquid long after the bottle is empty. Mary held the personified Christ, Love and Strength Itself, in her blessed womb for nine months before He entered into this world. She still to this day and forever will radiate the light of Love and Strength in her most beloved womb; this is why it is essential for us warriors to be her children and to be "re-formed"

> *"All my own perception of beauty in majesty and simplicity is founded upon Our Lady"*
> **— J.R.R. Tolkien.**

in the womb that bore Jesus, so that we might catch a small gasp of the delectable perfume that Mary brings into this miserable world. She is the moon and Jesus is the Sun, in which the moon gives light to the night, but not without the Sun.

Muslims have a devotion to her because even they can see the awesome power that she holds within her. She is the reason that Mexico had the conversion of millions of souls within a few years. Protestants envy her and think that we worship her because of our devotion. She is the heart and soul of all of Pope John Paul II's writings. She is the gates needed to pass through in order the reach the Way, the Truth and the Life. She is the oven that the bread of life was to rise within. Her blood flowed through God's veins. Her womb is what we need in order to be formed again as her Son, Jesus Christ was formed. She can only bring us closer to our Lord.

Pope Benedict XV hailed Mary as "Mother of the Prince of Peace, Mediatrix between rebellious man and merciful God... She is the dawn of peace shining in the darkness of a world out of joint; she never ceases to implore her Son for peace, although his hour is not yet come. She always intervenes on behalf of sorrowing humanity in the hour of danger. Today she, who is the mother of so many orphans and our advocate in this tremendous catastrophe, will most readily hear our prayers."

In St. Louis De Montfort's *True Devotion to the Blessed Virgin Mary* he invigorates us to fight for our beloved Queen, "Like every good servant and slave we must not remain idle, but, relying on her protection, we should undertake and carry out great things for our noble Queen. We must defend her privileges when they are questioned and uphold her good name when it is under attack. We must attract everyone, if possible, to her service and to this true and sound devotion. We must speak up and denounce those who distort devotion to her by outraging her Son, and at the same time we must apply ourselves to spreading this true devotion. As a reward for these little services, we should expect nothing in return save the honor of belonging to such a lovable Queen and the joy of being united through her to Jesus, her Son, by a bond that is indissoluble in time and in eternity. Glory to Jesus in Mary! Glory to Mary in Jesus! Glory to God alone!"[4] Mary is constantly under attack by the secular world, whether it be artwork with her picture on it accompanied by human dung (I do not joke about this, check out Bill Donohue's *Secular Sabotage*, to read up on the worst of it), or music videos showing her as a promiscuous, sleazy woman, we must question why it is that Mary is the person who many non-believers and many people who thoroughly hold disdain for our queen dislike her. We must stand up for her honor.

> *In St. Louis de Montfort's True Devotion to the Blessed Virgin Mary he states, "Mary is the supreme masterpiece of Almighty God and he has reserved the knowledge and possession of her for himself. She is the glorious Mother of God the Son who chose to humble and conceal her during her lifetime in order to foster her humility.... No creature, however pure, may enter there without being specially privileged."*

Mary is the perfect model of the precision of obedience to her reason and the will of the Father. As we discipline our bodies to follow our minds and wills through the art of lifting weights or exercise, pushing ourselves to the limit of exhaustion, we can tell our bodies who is really in command. We will put our lower nature in its place and allow our reason and conscience to take control. In

Thomas Aquinas' *Shorter Summa* he says, "So, in the Blessed Virgin Mary the sensitive (sensual) appetite was rendered so subject to reason by the power of the grace which sanctified it that it was never aroused against reason but always conformed to the order of reason." We must look to our heavenly Mother as our model to never surrender to temptation and train our minds, bodies, and souls to be in faultless conformity to the will of God. Without Mary it is safe to say that the salvation of the world would never have taken place. God can obviously do whatever He wishes but Mary is the beginning of our salvation history, without her there is no end. Father Donald Calloway in a talk on the relationship between Mary and the *Theology of the Body* explains that Mary is our ultimate goal; she is the only human to ever reach the pinnacle of love and devotion to God through her mind, body and soul most perfectly. Our Catholic faith is known as the Marian Church because we put her on such a high pedestal, and rightfully so. Mary is our perfect model of cheerful obedience and the realization that our bodies are gifts to be given back in love.

> **"Let the storm rage and the sky darken - not for that shall we be dismayed. If we trust as we should in Mary, we shall recognize in her, the Virgin Most Powerful 'who with virginal foot did crush the head of the serpent"**
> **— Pope St. Pius X**

Suggested Prayer

Mary, our most perfect and Immaculate Mother, I give everything I am and have to your most holy service. Let me never weary from my duties as your soldier and always keep me close to your heart. Crush the head of Satan and his many minions that lurk through this world. Please, my lady, bring me closer to your Son. Before the end of the day pray the rosary.

V

Thou shalt use this time to appreciate what masculinity is — truly a gift from The Almighty

'That night I asked the Mother of God what was to become of me.
Then she came to me holding two crowns, one white, the other red.
She asked if I was willing to accept either of these crowns.
The white one meant that I should persevere in purity,
and the red that I should become a martyr.
I said that I would accept them both.'

—Maximilian Kolbe

What is a man? The dictionary defines man as "A male human endowed with qualities, such as strength, considered characteristic of manhood." When does a boy enter into manhood? What makes a man willing to fight and die for something he believes in? Why does our society seem to have a real lack or misunderstanding of what makes a true man? Where have all the real men gone? These are the questions that are facing our world today. As many men, I'm sure, grew up watching John Wayne, or Superman and dreamed of one day being able to step up and take these men's places for the next generation. When I was a boy I would look to these examples and be invigorated to be like them and then came the teenager years. As I entered into my teens I started realizing, or the world told me, that these types of men were mostly fictional characters and that most men could never reach that high of a goal or potential. My father is a masculine and honorable man, one day I hope to be as spiritually strong and disciplined as he is. But when you are growing up in a culture that tells you that your fathers are not your examples and to instead look to the latest rock star or movie star where does one end up looking? As most of us men can say, in the realm of sex, drugs, and rock and roll. Our society tells us that this is where the "real" men are at. There is the type of man that would kill you as soon as look at you, the womanizer, or the metro-sexual fashion model as the examples that the world offers young men to emulate. I fell somewhere in between the womanizer and the tough guy. The more I searched for a real man the harder they were to find, in the secular world that is. A boy dreams about growing up and being that knight in shining armor that slays the dragon and wins the damsel in distress. Unfortunately this idea is abandoned somewhere along the way either because of self-pity, lack of confidence, or outside sources of sin such as pornography, bad music, or many other sources. So what is a real man and where can we find Him? This question has one answer: Jesus Christ.

Because of today's mega-church attitude the idea that Jesus was more of a moral teacher rather than a savior and a martyr for the only cause worth dying for has caused many men to stray away from the idea of faith. We have to realize who and what Jesus was as a man in order for all men to really appreciate His masculinity. To do so one only has to open up the Gospels. In Luke 4:28–30 it says, "When they heard this, the entire synagogue was filled with wrath. And they rose up and put Him out of the city, and led Him to a brow of the hill on which their city was built, that they might throw Him down headlong. But passing through the midst of them He went away." Jesus was in essence being attacked by an angry mob that was intent on killing, or viciously wounding Him because of the teachings that He was spreading. The world does not know how to react to chaste masculine love and it is always attacked by anger. This is a great example of a real man. A fire and pitchfork mob dragged Him to a cliff and He simply got up and walked right through them.

The ability to stare your enemy in the eye with a weapon as great as love is real power. A real man is unafraid of attack and unafraid to speak the truth to the masses. A real man has a presence about Him. This is very similar to the magnetism that one feels when around a pregnant woman, they give off a presence, which causes people to look in awe at the person. This glow that we see is the fulfillment of the feminine duties and abilities which are God given, bringing the image and likeness of God to the world. So when Jesus walked through the angry mob that day it was the fundamental nature of a real man that caused the people to let Him go. It reminds me of a story of St. Francis, he was walking to an area that was filled with Moors, or Muslims, who were known for killing Christians, because of the essence that illuminated off of him the Moors were afraid to touch him.

Part of the ill-defined mode of manliness in our world today is that boys no longer are pushed to have heroes. Boys grow up today watching Spongebob Squarepants instead of Superman, they read about mischievous little wizards rather than the knight saving the damsel in distress. The world tells them to follow your own conscience and forget what others think, which is ok in its own right if the conscience is properly formed, but there is a need to have a hero to look up to and want to imitate. A real hero is one who sacrifices himself for the greater cause, just as Jesus did. Many saints and many great men have fought on the battlefields, whether spiritual or corporal, and died for something greater than he. There is a reason that stories of warfare and fighting to the end touch the heart of every boy, it is precisely because this way of life, a sacrificial one, is what we are all called to. Even for non-Christians Jesus Christ's death can be viewed as a masculine one. People who do not believe in the message of the Gospel can still recognize the sacrifice this Man gave for what He believed in. Not to mention the fact that Jesus dragged a 200-250 lb. cross for quite a ways and up a hill while the crowds were spitting and throwing rocks at Him, while He had a crown of thorns on His head, and in addition had almost every inch of flesh stripped off of His body, can attest to the fact that this Man was a real man.

Jesus gave us an excellent example of how to live out that knight in shining armor lifestyle. Rather than shining armor He was covered in the armor of blood, and He defeated the dragon (Satan) by sacrificing Himself for our sins, and saved the damsel in distress, His beloved bride, The Catholic Church, by the Throne of the cross. If young boys and young men started seeing this man's man as an example to live by rather than what the world offers, we would have an end to pornography, birth control, abortion, effeminate lifestyles, injustice, corruption, and many other sins that good men are falling into. Regrettably, the secular world does not offer young men true heroes of Christ-like quality. In the documentary *Bigger, Stronger, Faster* one of Chris Bell's brothers says, "I'd rather die than be normal", I think that this statement helps exemplify how young men feel these days, our 'heroes' we look up to are anything but normal, and we are meant for greatness, but the normalcy of our heroes today are far away from the virtuous and magnanimous men and women we regard as saints. Without an example to live by how can we breed our sons into real men? By teaching them what virtue is and the proper application of each.

"Manliness is teachable."
— Euripides 423 B.C

The word virtue comes from the Greek expression virtus. This word literally means manliness, strength, toughness, simplicity, and bearing up against adversity. There are many virtues that can make a man but the cardinal virtues or 'hinge' virtues are the ones I wish to delve into. Obviously the virtues of faith, hope and love are extremely important but these are for another book. The four cardinal virtues are prudence, fortitude, temperance, and justice. "Which four virtues are called cardinal; for by prudence, we obey; by justice, we bear ourselves manfully; by temperance, we tread the serpent underfoot; by fortitude, we earn the grace of God" — St. Thomas Aquinas (Catena Aurea).

Prudence is an additional way to say the word wisdom. Our God who is wisdom itself gives man a taste of the knowledge that he contains. There is a difference between intelligence and wisdom. Many people can spatter out a few bible verses and pretend that they know the message of the gospels, but, real wisdom is shown in life application. If we do not know how to use these 'smarts' then what use are they?[2] Real wisdom is being able to know what is right and wrong and how to apply those things to real life, something the Church has perfected. As Bishop Fulton Sheen said in his book *Peace of Soul*, "There is a world of difference between knowing about God through study and knowing God through love — as great as the difference between a courtship carried on by mail and one by personal contact. Many skeptical professors know the proofs of the existence of God better than some who say their prayers; but because the professors never acted on the knowledge that they had, because they never loved God Whom they knew by study, no new knowledge of God was given to them. They liked to *talk* about religion but *did* nothing about it, and their knowledge remained sterile as a result." During the days of the early church it was the wise that made the world change, just as they do today, but without proper study and application we can never achieve our mission.

> **G. K. Chesterton once wrote, "To become Catholic is not to leave off thinking but to learn how to think."**

The second cardinal virtue is fortitude or courage. Marcus Cicero repeatedly stated that fortitude is the virtue that defines a real man, 'viri autem propria maxime est fortitudo'. When saints like Maximilian Kolbe or Thomas More are willing and able to step up and sacrifice their lives for something they believe in this takes courage. A man can apply bravery to his everyday life. A father that goes to work every day for his family, this takes valor, or the young man who says no to all the sins of the world for the one true God displays daring. When boys grow up bravery is part of the fabric of their lives. We are willing to climb trees as tall as a house and build a fort with no concern for the reality of the danger. We take part in swordfights and gun battles as if it were an everyday occurrence, knowing that what we were putting our lives on the line for was good and true. Disappointingly, somewhere along the way we lose sight of this sense of adventure and unpolluted principles. As we grow into young men we allow the reality of the world to set in and bury that heart deep down inside of us and set it in shackles. However, the Catholic Church has given us opportunity to take back that heart which is rightfully given to us by God. In the course of our spiritual growth we can take each occasion to grow in holiness leading to a truly audacious life. We must take back what God has given us and never let it be taken away again.

In St. Francis De Sales book, *The Love of God*, he defines temperance repressing the rebellious movements of sensuality. In other words it is the ability to suppress our lower nature with discipline and prayer. Temperance can also be classified as self-control. The high merit that willpower has for a man is endless. Healing an addiction takes willpower fused with plenty of prayer. With the overabundance of material in today's world that we have to get addicted to, temperance is the answer. This is where I believe lifting weights can in reality heal many of our addictions. If we have a problem eating too much, we can restrain ourselves. If we have a dependence on cigarettes, caffeine or pain pills we can push through. If one is obsessed with pornography we can allow our reason and will to be determined to overcome. Temperance combined with prayer and a sacramental life is a dangerous tool for us Catholics.

> **Pope Benedict XVI said at the Opening Mass of the 11th Ordinary General Assembly of the Synod of Bishops that, "nowhere that the human being makes himself the one lord of the world and owner of himself can justice exist. There, it is only the desire for power and private interests that can prevail."**

Lastly is the virtue that has appeared to lose its true meaning today, that is Justice. Many of the early Christians used the word justice in exchange for the word holiness. As citizens of today we think of justice as the blindfolded woman holding the scales, but I believe that the earlier generations of Catholics have a different outlook on this virtue. We seem to think of justice as a "to each his own" mentality and sometimes forget that our absolute reason for life is to give God the justice that is due to Him. When we think of justice today we tend to think that I deserve what I have worked for, which is good in its own right but not essentially the definition of justice. God is justice personified and His stance of fairness is so much deeper than our own, we think that our murderers deserve life in prison or worse, whereas our heavenly Father says that the murderer deserves love and affection. We have to take our sense of righteousness and fuse it with mercy and then we will begin to scratch the surface of true justice. The virtues are something that every man by necessity put to practice by daily habit. When we exercise or lift weights we can look into our own lives and contemplate on what virtues we are lacking in and search deep into our souls through the physical body and allow that God-given heart of a lion to come forth and force us to begin a daily routine of examination.

God, in His limitless intelligence, has endowed men and women with different hormones that define who we are sexually. Men have been given testosterone and women, estrogen and progesterone. Our civilization has caused men to think of testosterone as an animalistic hormone that is appalling and dangerous and therefore we should try and avoid it at all costs. This could not be further from the truth. Because of our feminized society, men are expected to be "nice guys" who just let everybody get along and never judge people's actions. If a man is too straight forward or too intense they need to go to, as Tim Staples once put it, sensitivity training, because there is something deeply wrong with that man. But if we are going to deny the very essence of who we are then we might as well deny the reality of evil in the world. We have to realize that our boys for at least the last two generations have been raised like women. Male children are told never to fight, don't jump in the mud, and please just get along with everyone, which is a feminine modality of life. The term "boys will be boys" is now looked upon as a negative thing. In a book named *The Art of Manliness* by Brett McKay, I think he said it best when he wrote, "Discouraged from celebrating the positive aspects of manliness, society today focuses only on the stereotypical and negative aspects of manhood. Sadly, manliness has come to be associated with the dithering dads of television sitcoms and commercial, the shallow action of dudes of cinema who live to blow stuff up and the meatheads of men's magazines who covet six-pack abs above all else ... The art of manliness just needs to be rediscovered."

While boys are growing up they naturally want to learn how to fight and how far their strength can take them. Boys are born with a natural want for conflict and adventure. James Stenson stated that when boys are born they will look into the eyes of the person holding them for a couple seconds and then start to look around, whereas girls will keep eye contact for much longer, boys are meant for adventure and girls are meant for relationships. Now I am not saying that all boys need to get in

> **"Cowards die many times before their deaths; the valiant never taste of death but once."**
> **— William Shakespeare**

fights or conquer the world, but if a boy does not learn to stand up for themselves or go take that possibly dangerous step at some age, they never will. This, I believe is why the pornography, abortion, and homosexual movements have all gotten as far as they have, because men are not willing to take a stand and say, "No more!"

If a boy is never shown how to swallow fear and face it like a man, then they never will, and evil will prevail. "Manliness consists not in bluff, bravado or lordliness. It consists in daring to do the right and facing consequences whether it is in matters social, political or other. It consists in deeds, not in words"— Gandhi. Testosterone is a man's physical engine to stand up and fight when nobody else will, just as the Holy Spirit is our spiritual engine.

In the *Theology of the Body*, Pope John Paul II, defines men and women mostly by what they were at the beginning of creation, before human beings contained the stain of sin. By means of the same rationale we can securely proclaim that Adam, before the fall of man, was in complete control and aware of his masculinity, which includes his testosterone. With Adam encompassing perfect masculinity God gives Adam the task of naming the animals and putting him in the wilderness to figure himself out before He could ever allow man to meet woman. There is a dire need in a man's soul to work with his hands and be part of the rough country. Our eyes see a remarkable landscape or horizon and our hearts leap in our chests. For instance, I remember growing up and my family and I would be driving on a vacation somewhere and my mother would always get frustrated with my father because he would be looking around at construction or some type of landscape and 'wouldn't be paying attention to the road'. And I have to say I am guilty of the same habit, and my wife would very quickly agree. Nevertheless, it is because of our masculinity that our hearts desire to see these things, we see a mountainside or a cliff and begin to think on how we would scale it. We see construction and start wondering which type and brand of tools they are using to build with. I believe that lifting weights and exercise is a healthy and equitable mode of reaching into our masculine spirit and transporting it to the fore front.

Men's hands are intended to be rough and to be in contact with coarse materials. It feels good to a man to grab a hammer or some steel. What better way to express that love of unforgiving steel than hitting the weight room? I remember when I had my first real experience of the beauty of lifting weights. I was a junior in high school when I started lifting on my own and one day I grabbed the bar in order to complete my last set of bench and just sat there for a moment grazing my hand across that cold and ruthless steel and I was hooked. I didn't grow up in a family of hunters; my father is an extremely masculine man nonetheless. He helped me to understand how a man must push himself to greatness and never to surrender through his love of God and His Church, and the weight room. I was a rebellious teenager and at the time the physical world was all that I cared about, I had a deep respect for God and The Catholic Church, but I was selfish. Later in my life when I finally decided to take hold of my masculinity and become the Catholic man that God creates all men to be, I united my love of lifting with my love of God and from there my fight against temptation has never been the same. When I feel stressed or in need of some prayer time I am able mix the physicality of lifting, something that makes sense to men in the corporal realm, with the splendor of prayer.

This method of prayer reminds me of the warrior monks of the Crusades, such as the Knights Templar, who mastered the skills of their bodies and sharpened the proficiency of their souls to the degree that their pious devotion to the Faith is unrivaled. These were the chief warriors that the Muslims had fear of and their legends are still dreamed of today. The combining of the physical and spiritual permitted these soldiers for God to have no qualms over fighting and dying for the Faith. In the Catholic Encyclopedia under the history of the All Hallow College, an Irish all men's school devoted to philosophy, Catholicism, ethics, etc. the encyclopedia stated that part of the regimen for the students to learn was, "They are also encouraged to develop health and *manliness* by outdoor exercises and recreations, such as football, hurling, hockey, handball, tennis, cricket, athletic competitions, and long walks." (Italics added) The weight room can become our monasteries. Men need to put themselves through hardships because this is how we get closer to God. Men are physical beings and we have a heavenly obligation to foster and cherish our mortality.

In Frank Miniter's book The Ultimate Man's Survival Guide he states, "Men need to be well rounded. But ignoring this (physical) part of an education can leave a man without the physical confidence earned from the toil and triumph of competition. This is why the Greeks used sport to teach a boy to push his body, to take his stamina to new limits. They saw it as training for battle and manhood. They knew the human body is capable of much more than someone who has never really pushed their body realizes. It's a necessary step on the path to manhood to harness the confidence and self-knowledge that comes from this understanding of one's body. Whether big or small, strong or weak, young or old, a person who has learned what his body can and can't do is more likely to tackle life's conflicts with quiet confidence — and that is manly."

Jesus had a very strong sense of His masculinity, and he wasn't afraid to do what was needed. He would go to the Pharisees and call them out in front of the whole town if they were doing wrong, the Pharisees would be comparable to politicians or teachers today so it would have been quite an odd ordeal to correct them in their thinking. He even called Peter, the future leader of His church, Satan at one point because he was in the way of Jesus completing His mission. If we are called to be like Jesus then men must go back to having a real sense of who they are as strong, masculine men. Jesus did not come to bring peace; he came to bring division between the good and the wicked. He wasn't worried about everyone "getting along" and not judging people by their actions. When Jesus told His followers, before the institution of the Eucharist, that unless we eat His flesh and drink His blood we have no life within us half the people left. He didn't call those people back, He simply let them go. I could write an entire book on manliness and Jesus' unrelenting masculine mind-set, but I will leave you with this, in Fr. Larry Richards' book, *Be a Man!*, he says, "This is not the time to be a wimp! Today the world needs real men! Your family is counting on you; your friends are counting on you; your world is counting on you; your God is counting on you- so don't be afraid: take courage and be a man!"

Suggested Prayer

My Lord, I surrender my life to you, but especially this day my corporal body in order that it be most perfectly utilized by You. I long to be your servant, your soldier, and your martyr, and I know that without proper training I cannot fulfill my duties. Good St. Joseph teach me to use my hands like a man, help me to desire a rich understanding of my role as a man. Jesus was given to you because you were a confident, magnanimous male; teach me as you taught our Lord.

Amen

VI

Thou shalt never use this time for Self-glorification — vanity is deadly

"Vanity is so secure in the heart of man that everyone wants to be admired: even I who write this, and you who read this."

– *Blaise Pascal*

It can be said that all sins lead back to pride. The original sin of our first parents was a result of the want to be like God. With our current society the want to be recognized and glorified is so unbelievably rampant. Our gyms are filled with mirrors on every side so that we can check ourselves out while we lift just to bask in our own greatness. The women in our tabloids and magazines have so much plastic surgery that they sometimes don't even look human anymore. Vanity is an extremely deadly and contagious problem that must be amended if we can ever have a selfless and truly Christian society. Never before in human history has vanity been this unrestrained and admired. Don't get me wrong, I think each and every human being should try and make themselves as beautiful as possible because we are all God's children and therefore owe it to Him to keep ourselves at our pinnacle, but if beauty is worth more than our souls then there is a serious problem. God has decided to make us in His image and likeness and therefore we do have something to be particularly proud of.

We have the desire in all of us to better ourselves in mind, body and soul. "I *deserve* better than this!" Sound familiar? We have this innate want to have the things that we think are going to make us happy, one of which is a perfect body. Our culture today causes people that want to look better desire perfection. Not only perfection but rapidly acquired perfection. When we see the people in the limelight that have these perfect bodies and seem so unbelievably happy we only need to look at their personal lives and realize that they are not. Have you ever seen a professional bodybuilder in the off-season? They have acne everywhere, fat hanging off of them, and look absolutely miserable. Why is it that we look up to these people?

"I recognized that there is nothing better than to be glad and to do well during life. For every man, moreover, to eat and drink and enjoy the fruit of all his labor is a gift of God" (Ecclesiastes 3:12 –13).

Ecclesiastes gives first-rate examples of the accurate mode of self-appreciation. This quote from chapter 3 gives a definition of why it is that we want better things in this world, and how our world distorts this definition. When we lift weights or exercise our desire should be to improve ourselves for the greater glory of God. So what is the difference between self-appreciation and vanity? Look at the quote above, what is the main word in the verse? The answer is: God. We must keep Him in our sights when we aspire to better ourselves, without Him it surely will be vanity driving us to excel. As much as I disagree with Ayn Rand's atheist point of view, in her book *The Virtue of Selfishness* she illustrates my point very well. "If a man's values are such that he desires things which, in fact and in reality, lead to his destruction, his emotional mechanism will not save him, but will, instead, urge him on toward destruction: he will have set it in reverse, against himself and against the facts of reality, against his own life." What this is saying is that the values that we choose to follow will decide the outcome of our hard work. If our values are based off of the need to be praised and glorified we will lean towards our own demise because men are not, by human nature, to be glorified as given by the example of Jesus Christ. If we desire to glorify God and everyone else in Christian charity, the end result of our hard work will lead us to the divine nature in which God desires to give us. So, when we have the want to have better health and a better appearance I am in complete belief that this desire comes from the Almighty and that it is what we do with this craving that will define the outcome. If we want to be happy and healthy we must include a sacrificial lifestyle or else we aspire to make ourselves better through selfish desires which will cause our own lives to crash down upon us. How can we keep ourselves in the pursuit of bodily perfection while remaining humble and reasonable?

> *"Follow the ways of your heart, the vision of your eyes; yet understand that as regards all this, God will bring you to judgment"* *(Ecclesiastes 11:9).*

Vanity is synonymous with vainglory. The definition of vainglory is honor given to a person not based on reality or reason. So with common sense one could easily say that vanity is based off of an emptiness or futility. We cannot take the fame, the fortune, or the glory with us to the afterlife. Man struggles with this thought as did Dorian Gray "How sad it is! I shall grow old, and horrid, and dreadful. But this picture will remain always young. It will never be older than this particular day of June … If it was only the other way! If it was I who were to be always young, and the picture that were to grow old! For this — for this — I would give everything! Yes, there is nothing in the whole world I would not give!" — *The Picture of Dorian Gray* by Oscar Wilde. Satan wants us to think that we are going to be around forever, just as he tempted Adam and Eve, and many times while in the pursuit of health and better bodily image we try and justify our thoughts of immortality. I think The Picture of Dorian Gray gives an excellent example of how far we will try to keep that image of ourselves that we most enjoy. But, what would eternal life be without God, miserable. When we strive for the betterment of our health or body image we have to keep in mind that we are mortal beings and that without God we would not be able to take our next breath. When the pain of one more repetition or the grief of denying ourselves that after-dinner ice cream sets in we must decide then and there, this is where we can benefit from the taste of our own mortality and realize how much we depend on God's grace and blessings. The search for immortality is only fulfilled in the light of the Cross. If we do not want to suffer for our eternal reward here on earth we will suffer for eternity. Just as guilty pleasure is revoked through innocent suffering, so vanity is rescinded through humility. Being humble is what makes men great. The late Archbishop Fulton Sheen stated that, "There are two types of people that Jesus came for, the people who do not know anything and those who understand enough to know that they do not know everything." Without humility we can achieve nothing because without humility one does not have God within their heart, and without God nothing is possible. Humility is a necessity of growth and without it the spirit of a man is stifled.

As men, humility is a difficult concept to completely define. We want to be humble yet we also do not want to be stepped on. We have the urge to protect those around us and also to want the respect of others, so when we strive for a humble lifestyle it is difficult to deny the internal need for admiration. Where is the line drawn between glory and humility? Robert E. Lee once stated that "A true man of honor feels humbled himself when he cannot help humbling others." A masculine man has the innate ability to humble those around him without ever becoming conscious of the fact that he does. I will never forget when I met Francis Cardinal Arinze it was very difficult to not look at him with awe and respect before he ever said a word. He carried himself as a man should and therefore he gets treated like a man but all the while he is the most loving and kind man one could meet.

Being humble does not mean that we must grovel in cowardice of those who wish to do us harm. Meekness should never be confused with the kind of person that allows cruelty or any such disgrace to continue. Meekness is the ability to stay strong in the face of malice to oneself and not to rise in anger, however in the presence of moral tyranny to others we are required to take action. Jesus was perfectly humble yet shook the earth to its core by being a man willing to lay His life on the line to the point of death on a cross. George Washington has always been depicted as a humble and considerate man yet when he decided to speak an entire room would be silenced by the utterance of his words. The Holy Spirit is the object of desire if one wishes to be humble yet not fragile. When a man is filled with the Holy Spirit he can take on the world.

People might ask me "So how does a person try and perfect his body without increasing in vanity? That seems impossible!" While this task is daunting and not for the weak of heart, it is not impossible. St. Francis de Sales, in his book *Introduction to the Devout Life* he stated "There is no fear that a perception of what He has given you will puff you up, so long as you keep steadily in mind that whatever is good in you is not of yourself." As images of Divine Beauty our striving for perfection is a call from our Artist. Vain thoughts will come and go nevertheless our struggle to suppress the egoism in all of us will bring us closer to the heart of God. Allowing Him into our hearts as we exercise our bodies will allow the paintbrush of our Almighty Father to smother our souls in grace. "On the contrary, a lively appreciation of the grace given to you should make you humble,

"Do you not know that your body is a temple of the Holy Spirit within you, whom you have from God, and that you are not your own? For you have been purchased at a price. Therefore, glorify God in your body"
(1 Corinthians 6:19-20).

for appreciation begets gratitude. But if, when realizing the gifts God has given you, any vanity should beset you; the infallible remedy is to turn to the thought of all our ingratitude, imperfection, and weakness. Anyone who will calmly consider what he has done without God, cannot fail to realize that what he does with God is no merit of his own; and so we may rejoice in that which is good in us, and take pleasure in the fact, but we shall give all the glory to God Alone, Who Alone is its Author" (*Introduction to the Devout Life*).

When we decide to take the challenge of following God with our mind, body and soul we must consider the fact that our body is the tool of which our mind and soul uses to prove our loyalty. A father does not prove his love from thoughts or words to his children; he confirms his affections through his actions and genuine physical contact with them. Any good deed that is done through our bodies not only glorifies God but glorifies our own bodies. This is a reciprocal relationship. While we perform charitable acts out of love of God and love of neighbor we receive the grace from God to continue the acts which allows our bodies to continue to glorify The Almighty. If we did not have mouths to speak we could not spread the Good News. If we did not have ears we could not listen to the needs of our people. If we did not have hands our priests could not complete the Holy Sacrifice of the altar. Vanity would only destroy any of the good that comes from these charitable acts. It is the same principle in the weight room. While we are venerating God through the improvement of our bodies we allow the grace of pleasing God to enter into our souls, if we allow pride to take hold of our deed we cut off the channel from which God can disperse that grace.

For the closing prayers, I would like to leave you with a thought from Thomas A. Kempis' *Imitation of Christ*. He beautifully describes the relationship between grace and vanity.

> "Thanks be to Thee, from whom all cometh, whensoever it goeth well with me! But I am vanity and nothing in Thy sight, a man inconstant and weak. What then have I whereof to glory, or why do I long to be held in honour? Is it not for nought? This also is utterly vain. Verily vain glory is an evil plague, the greatest of vanities, because it draweth us away from the true glory, and robbeth us of heavenly grace. For whilst a man pleaseth himself he displeaseth Thee; whilst he gapeth after the praises of man, he is deprived of true virtues. But true glory and holy rejoicing lieth in glorying in Thee and not in self; in rejoicing in Thy Name, not in our own virtue; in not taking delight in any creature, save only for Thy sake. Let thy Name, not mine be praised; let Thy work, not mine be magnified; let Thy holy Name be blessed, but to me let nought be given of the praises of men. Thou art my glory; Thou art the joy of my heart. In Thee will I make my boast and be glad all the day long, for myself let me not glory save only in my infirmities."

- Thomas A Kempis

VII

Thou shalt pray before, during, and after one lifts

"I prayed for twenty years but received no answer until I prayed with my legs."

Frederick Douglass, escaped slave

Fulton Sheen once said, "Why should we pray? Why breathe? We have to take in fresh air and get rid of bad air; we have to take in new power and get rid of old weaknesses. We pray because we are orchestras and always need to tune-up. Just as a battery sometimes winds down and needs to be charged, so we have to be renewed in spiritual vigor." Prayer is what makes the heart yearn for something better. It is incredible to me how much our bodies can tell us about our souls. We must constantly die to ourselves spiritually so that we can become closer to God. As St. Augustine said, "I must decrease so that He may increase." So it is with our bodies. In order for more muscle to grow we must tear down the old muscles, which will cause us pain, but in the end we will be much better for it. Prayer is what causes this type of reaction for the soul. It lets our ego get out of the way and open wide the doors of our heart for Christ. If we do not pray we do not grow in our relationship to a loving God. When we look at some of the most holy people that ever walked this earth, Mother Teresa for example, we tend to look at the physical part of their being. Mother Teresa was a small and dainty person, yet when one thinks of how much power her prayer possessed, she is a massive giant. Our prayer lives must be the heart of our personal relationship with our Trinitarian God. We are the Church militant and so, as would parents who have their children off at war, God wants as much correspondence as He can get from us. I believe that if we can combine the spiritual power of prayer with the physical power of lifting weights and exercise we can become a dangerous adversary to the devil.

Anyone who has ever seriously lifted weights or even just once in their lifetime can recall a specific period of time just before you grab the bar or dumbbell, there is a time there when you start to think of what you are about to do. Your life can flash before your eyes and all of your worries can dissipate, because at that very moment you are about to go to war with yourself. Now, I ask, what better time in life is there to say a prayer? Before all of the great wars of this world there was a send-off speech by a great general or officer. "What we do in life echoes in eternity!" is a great line from the movie *Gladiator* that I think illustrates my point. Before a man is lead into battle, and we as Catholics are already at war, he needs an ending thought in his mind in order to remember what it is he is fighting for. We are not fighting for anything that this world can offer; instead we fight for a cause that only God Himself can propose. Just before you step up to the weights you can remind yourself that, "What we do in life echoes in eternity!" and declare to yourself, to the underworld and to God Himself that you are a man and you are here to fight. This type of prayer is what a man's soul longs for, and unless you are a soldier in an earthly battle, we men are not given too many chances to reach this type of desire. This is how combining lifting and prayer will fill that void.

St. Benedict said it best when he stated "He who labors as he prays lifts his heart to God with his hands." He was speaking to his monastic brothers when he made this statement that flows perfectly with his motto of "Ora et labora" or "Pray and work". He was addressing the labor that his monasteries were to do, farming, house chores, etc. For the purpose of this book I want to take his statement and bring it into our current topic. Hard labor is considered by St. Benedict as one of the highest means of sanctification. In the same way we can make the corporal labor of lifting weight into a means of holiness. The union between our souls and our bodies is so intimate that we can participate in the spiritual through the physical and vice versa. So, when we pray while we lift the labor of our hands and muscles are united to that prayer. Our prayers are brought to God and so therefore our muscles and sweat become the means to which we offer our prayers to God. This extends to the consideration that when we lift and pray our very lives, physical and spiritual, are given back to our loving Creator.

This reminds me of the beauty of incense used during mass. We use the physical nature of heat and incense to present our prayers to God. We burn the incense so that it may rise to God, we smell the incense to enliven our senses, we see the smoke rising to the heavens, reminding us of the Divine Nature we long for, and we hear the clank of the chain as the priest swings the thurible. In the same way we burn our muscles so that they may rise to God, we smell our body working to enliven our senses, we see the sweat falling off of our bodies, reminding us of our mortality, and we hear the clank of steel as we lift. Our gyms can truly become our monasteries if we beg, pray, and allow God to take control of the experience. Prayer is such an essential part of our lives; we must take it into the weight room with us.

> *"**PRAYER** opens the understanding to the brightness of Divine Light, and the will to the warmth of Heavenly Love, nothing can so effectually purify the mind from its many ignorance's, or the will from its perverse affections. It is as healing water which causes the roots of our good desires to send forth fresh shoots, which washes away the soul's imperfections, and allays the thirst of passion*
> *— Francis De Sales Intro to the Devout Life.*

We would not go a whole day without trying to eat something to nourish our bodies and such it is with the soul. When we do not feed it with the spiritual sustenance of prayer to our Creator we become like starving little children scrounging around a dump heap looking for something to fill our bellies. Our bodies are at war with our souls, our corporal being tends to lean toward worldliness, while our souls hunger for the love of God. Without a devotion to prayer and a regular prayer life, the darkness of this world will be severely difficult to overcome in times of trial and hardship. Without a daily practice of lifting up our bodies and souls to the Almighty we will fail to do so in times of difficulty. Now, if we were to practice a prayer life during habitual, voluntary, physical suffering, along with our absolute necessity of daily prayers, we can ourselves have souls of a lions. I was recently asked what our reactions are to be if say we were in Nazi Germany and was asked to deny our faith in order to save our lives and the possibility of saving others lives. If we desire a crown of martyrdom then the answer is to say, "I am a Catholic and I will not deny my King, Jesus Christ!" with such boldness and confidence that we shake the very halls of hell. If we were to ever come face to face with such persecution, would it be easier to say something of the sort with or without a habitual prayer life and a daily offering of our voluntary, physical anguish? I am fully convinced that if we are to put ourselves through a daily routine of pushing our bodies, all the while praying to God for more strength, we will triumph in the face of persecution.

Consistency breeds habits. When a person wants to change their life, either physically, mentally or spiritually, they must decide what needs to be done and accomplish this goal daily. If a liar wants to stop his habit of lying he must make a daily commitment to do so. It is the same with our prayer lives. We should strive to have certain habits that oblige us to repeatedly fall to our knees, day in and day out. For example, I have a hard time getting up early enough for my morning prayers, so I have put my alarm clock far enough away so that I have to get up in order to turn it off. By the time I have turned it off I am awake enough to pray. So it is with our physical lives, if we desire to better our health, we must put in place certain duties that must be accomplished daily.

History has given many examples of the power of prayer mixed with physical action. One of my favorites is in the Book of Joshua, specifically the battle of Jericho. God gave His commands as to how the Israelites were to pray and the actions that they were to take for 7 long days in order to defeat their enemies.

> "And to Joshua the LORD said, I have delivered Jericho
> and its king into your power. Have all the soldiers circle
> the city, marching once around it. Do this for six days, with
> seven priests carrying ram's horns ahead of the ark. On the
> seventh day march around the city seven times, and have
> the priests blow the horns. When they give a long blast on
> the ram's horns and you hear that signal, all the people shall
> shout aloud. The wall of the city will collapse, and they will
> be able to make a frontal attack" (Joshua 6: 2–5).

God didn't ask these warriors to lay low and try and pray maybe, if it isn't any trouble, to perhaps say one prayer for world peace. NO! He asked them to step up in the face of their adversaries and let them know that God is with us and we will prevail because of His righteousness. We are not meant to be fighters in the shadows, we are meant to be the voice of Faith to this broken world. How can we do that if we do not allow our prayer lives to be a dominant force in our relationship with others? Also, did you notice what God's intent was when the walls actually fall? *"And they will be able to make a frontal attack,"* He still intended for His people to go into the city and fight. He was not going to hand over a victory to His soldiers without their involvement. This is the true power of prayer. We beg and plead with God to help us on our earthly journey to take away our stumbling blocks and vices so that we can grow in holiness. But, in the end God will still expect us to fight. Why would a commander give his best weapon to a soldier that does not plan to use it?

A deepened sense of our dependence on God can intensify our prayer lives so that we will be able to achieve our goals in the weight room. Our prayers are more powerful than we could ever imagine. "Prayer gives us strength for great ideals, for keeping up our faith, charity, purity, generosity; prayer gives us strength to rise up from indifference and guilt, if we have had the misfortune to give in to temptation and weakness. Prayer gives us light by which to see and to judge from

"Look kindly on the prayer and petition of your servant, O LORD, my God, and listen to the cry of supplication your servant makes before you. May your eyes watch day and night over this temple, the place where you have decreed you shall be honored; may you heed the prayer which I your servant offer toward this place" (2 Chronicles 6:19–20).

God's perspective and from eternity. That is why you must not give up on praying!" (Pope John Paul II). Imagine yourself in a fortress. You feel that you are all alone and you can hear the rumblings of an oncoming army ready to devour you and destroy your stronghold. Each time you beg God for aid there suddenly appears a bowman. Each time you praise God for his goodness and mercy there appears a catapult. The more and more you pray, the more warriors and weapons appear on your side of the battlefield. Suddenly the oncoming assault seems to be much less fearsome. You know in your heart that a battle will still ensue but the more and more support you have the more confidence you have in your ability to fight. Our prayer lives are our method of living out a true warrior mentality. By mixing the spiritual nature of prayer with the physical nature of exercise we can create a process by which our Lord can fulfill that which is lacking in our own prayers.

Life is nothing without prayer. We must keep up our communication with our Lord in order to persistently grow in a loving relationship with Him. Many saints, such as St. Therese of Liseux, have perfected the ability to constantly be in contact with our Lord. First, we must learn how to pray, then we must continually do so, then we must learn how to unite it with our very lives. In closing I will leave you with a poem by one of my favorite authors. I believe this is what prayer should sound like.

A Hymn by G.K. Chesterton

O God of earth and altar, Bow down and hear our cry,

Our earthly rulers falter, Our people drift and die;

The walls of gold entomb us, The swords of scorn divide,

Take not thy thunder from us, But take away our pride.

From all that terror teaches, From lies of tongue and pen,

From all the easy speeches That comfort cruel men,

From sale and profanation Of honor and the sword,

From sleep and from damnation, Deliver us, good Lord.

Tie in a living tether The prince and priest and thrall,

Bind all our lives together, Smite us and save us all;

In ire and exultation Aflame with faith, and free,

Lift up a living nation, A single sword to thee.

VIII

Thou shalt pray that one's strength is useful in the will of God

'The dignity and power of this motive no man can fully comprehend; a single action, even the least and most insignificant, done with the view of pleasing God alone, and of glorifying Him, is worth infinitely more … than many actions in themselves of the greatest value and worth."

-Lorenzo Scupoli Spiritual Combat

There once was a man that was nearly invincible. Every day he would pray that his strength and virility would be pleasing to God. He was of herculean stature and fed his soul and mind as well as he fed his body. People from around the world would inquire how it is that he was in such god-like shape and able to defend his people with unseen ability. One day this man was tempted by the world, in which he fell, and in the blink of an eye his strength and talents were taken from him. As soon as God realized that the man was not using the talents He bestowed upon him in the way they were intended, God punished him by taking them away. Just as God took paradise from Adam and Eve for disobedience, so God took the strength from Samson. I need to pick on Samson one more time. His story reveals so much about how life can turn out for men. This man among men had it all, strength, good looks, and hair that could make a lion envious, but when his eyes turned from pleasing God to indulging in the pleasures of this world God allowed his chastisement.

Hikers would not go on a trek without a destination to reach. A mountain climber would not aim to stop half way up the peak. If we are to truthfully desire the pinnacle of our abilities in all things then there is a supreme necessity to discern whether or not decisions are in accord with the will of God. If we desire anything in our lives that is not in agreement with the will of God then we are digging our own grave and we desire in vain. God knows exactly what we need when we need it. If building up our strength and our health for any other reason than fulfilling the will of God, the newly begotten qualities could very easily lead to our downfall. The strength and purity of our physical goals are completely dependent on our desire to follow the will of God. What God wants should be what we want. His omniscience and omnipotence can guarantee that when we are in line with His desires for us our goals will be untainted by any waste.

An illustration of how we are able to fulfill the will of God in our lives is the same as us trying to figure out the best routine for our goals and what our body needs to grow while at the same time staying away from injury, overtraining, or under training. We set guidelines for ourselves so that we can stay within the parameters of reasonable exercise. A novice lifter should not walk into a gym and put 500 lbs on the bench press because that person is disposing himself to serious injury. On the other side of the issue, a healthy young man should not grab 1 lb dumbbells to workout with and expect any type of growth. The person needs to do his homework by reading up on muscle growth or good routines to use, or he should ask others who have done their homework what

The Catechism of the Catholic Church states that, "Man is sometimes confronted by situations that make moral judgments less assured and decision difficult. But he must always seriously seek what is right and good and discern the will of God expressed in divine law." #1787.

would be best for him in order to reach his strength and fitness goals. So it is with trying to fulfill the will of God. Unless we do our homework through study and prayer or look to examples (saints) who have lived out the lifestyle we are wanting to acquire then we will find ourselves in the pitfalls of the spiritual life which can lead to either injury (sin) or a lack of growth and knowledge.

If we desire to have real development of our bodies and our health then the need for God is a stipulation. "For all creatures before they existed, were possible, not by any created power, since no creature is eternal, but by the divine power alone, inasmuch as God could produce them into existence. Thus, as the production of a thing into existence depends on the will of God, so likewise it depends on His will that things should be preserved; for He does not preserve them otherwise than by ever giving them existence; hence if He took away His action from them, all things would be reduced to nothing," — Summa Theologica. If we do not take God's will into account during our striving for perfection "all things would be reduced to nothing." This statement of St. Thomas Aquinas coincides with the story of Samson very well. If we aspire to have better health or larger, stronger muscles then we must have reliance on the fact that "the production of a thing (*muscles*) … depends on the will of God."

Sorry to say but because of the modern culture of body worshippers and extreme health advocates, the idea of following the will of God has all but left the mind and heart of the exercise movement, if it was ever there to begin with. The stereotypes of 'meathead' and 'loonies' have permeated the thoughts of those who are outside of the bodybuilding world. However, we can change the labels of this culture by giving to it what is lacking, a vision of the divine. "The human body is in its own right, God's masterpiece in the order of visible creation. In the field of physical culture, the Christian concept needs to receive nothing from the outside, but has much to give" — Pope Pius XII. The Christian concept that Pope Pius XII was speaking of is outlined in Romans 12:2, "And be not fashioned according to this world: but be ye transformed by the renewing of your mind, and ye may prove what is the good and acceptable and perfect will of God." Once people start to realize that God wants us to be perfect then we can saturate the culture of bodybuilding and exercise with a want to follow God's will and a need to please Him. When modern bodybuilding first started to take shape, back in the glory days of Steve Reeves, people saw them as men trying to compensate for a lack of personality and authentic manliness. Unfortunately, most bodybuilders today have confirmed them in their thinking. We Christians can give the sport of bodybuilding and strength training a new perspective of God's role within our lives. We can help others appreciate that the desires in our hearts to become strong and capable are a calling from our Creator to tend to our bodies and keep them at their prime. We do this by following the command of Romans 12:2.

> **"Therefore, since Christ suffered in the flesh, arm yourselves also with the same attitude (for whoever suffers in the flesh has broken with sin), so as not to spend what remains of one's life in the flesh on human desires, but on the will of God"**
> **(1 Peter 4:1–2).**

Let us not forget that the Christian life is not supposed to be easy, neither is the life of a healthy person. It requires self control and prudence to be able to stay in good shape these days. Most of us have somewhat sedentary lifestyles, either because of office work or too much TV watching, but this can change decently easy. We just need to keep our eyes on the prize and allow the hardships of a prudent lifestyle to become part of who we are. By enduring the difficulty of keeping our bodies in shape and allowing the little bit of suffering that it takes we can keep our desires on those of God. Always remember that, '... it is not enough that you should will and do these things that are most pleasing to God... you must will and do them as being moved by Him and with the motive of simply pleasing Him' — Lorenzo Scupoli *Spiritual Combat*.

The will of God is stated by Jesus in Matthew 5:48 when He said, "Be perfect, just as your heavenly Father is perfect." This is not a suggestion as much as it seems to be a command. God desires that we reach the peak of our created existence. If we are to spend eternity with Him in heaven, perfection is a requirement. We are supposed long for and strive after perfection in all things, mind, body and soul. Perfection is reached when these three things are in line with a pure and suitable love of God. That innate need, especially prevalent in men, to prove ourselves worthy of something comes from this desire in our hearts to be perfect. God is calling each and every one of us to love Him more than ourselves and we prove this love by desiring to do His will. Socrates acknowledged that "The end of life is to be like God, and the soul following God will be like Him." Aligning ourselves with the superior and perfect will of God and knowing that the deep aspiration to prove ourselves is actually a calling from a loving Creator can bring us closer to the divine, which in turn can bring us closer to our heavenly reward.

In the Treatise on the Love of God, Book 8, Chapter 14, St. Francis de Sales establishes brilliantly how it is that we are supposed to determine whether or not we are following the will of God, "And even in matters of consequence we must be very humble, and not think to find God's will by force of examination and subtlety of discourse; but having implored the light of the Holy Spirit, applied our consideration to the seeking of his good-pleasure, taken the counsel of our director, and if appropriate, of two or three other spiritual persons, we must resolve and determine in the name of God, and not afterwards revoke or doubt our choice, but devoutly, peacefully, and firmly pursue and keep to it. And although the difficulties, temptations and the various circumstances which occur in the course of executing our design, might cause us some doubt as to whether we had made a good choice, we must remain firm, and not regard such things, but consider that if we had made another choice we might have been a hundred times worse; to say nothing of our not knowing whether it be God's will that we should be exercised in consolation or desolation, in peace or war. Once the resolution has been holily taken, we must never doubt of the holiness of carrying it out; for unless we fail it cannot fail. To act in another manner is a mark of great self-love, or of childishness, weakness and silliness of spirit."

Socrates also stated that "The shortest and surest way to live with honor in the world is to be in reality what we would appear to be; all human virtues increase and strengthen themselves by the practice and experience of them." This declaration flows perfectly with our need to fulfill the will of God. If we do not practice the things that bring us closely aligned with what God wants we will never know how to achieve the divine goals. Beyond a single doubt the want to follow God is indeed a virtuous practice and if we want to live with honor we must follow what Socrates believed. If we want to be holy then we must act like it. Left to our own desires and cravings we will surely be led down a path of destruction and sin, we do not know what is best for us no matter how much we think we do. Our purpose in life is to know, love and serve God. How can we serve Him if our wishes are not God's wishes? If we do not follow the will of God then we are only backsliding and are actually doing harm to the end goal of serving God. When we think that we can do it all without Him, even in spiritual matters, failure and unhappiness will be the only outcome.

"Not my will but thine be done" was the battle cry of our blessed Lord before he took on the test of his destiny to save the world. The completion of the will of His Father was the driving force behind our Lord during the most excruciating pain known to man. A life fulfilled by allowing ourselves to be completely submersed in only wanting what God wants can lead to an outpouring of world changing grace. In the end we have to remember that we are all going to die one day. We will be judged according to our fulfillment of the will of the Father. God doesn't care if you can lift 1000 pounds or only 100 pounds, what he cares about is whether or not you tried to fulfill His will with the strength he gave you. In my weight room at home, next to a Crucifix, I have a large 2 ft. by 3 ft. framed picture of *The Death of Socrates* painted by Jacques-Louis David, I have it there to remind me that God's will is more important than life and that if we must die in service of Him then so be it.

Suggested Prayer:

Most high, glorious God, let your light fill the shadows of my heart and grant me, Lord, true faith, certain hope, perfect love, awareness and knowing, that I may fulfill Your holy will.

-St. Francis of Assisi

IX

Thou shalt listen for the Whispers of God in this Time of Reflection

"They are the strong ones of the earth, the mighty food
for good or evil, those who know how to keep silence
when it is a pain and a grief to them;
those who give time to their own souls
to wax strong against temptation,
or to the powers of wrath
to stamp upon them their withering passage."

- Ralph Waldo Emerson

This excerpt from Mr. Emerson is a strong portrayal of the beauty of silence. In silence we become wiser and more in depth with our Creator. Our world is full of consistent noise and the hustle of everyday life can lead us away from the Divine. God has never been one to be a very loud Creator when conversing with His children, most of the time he uses others or the smallest 'whispers' to let us hear what we need to, which is as it should be. If anyone were to hear the full blown voice of Our Lord, that person would die on the spot as our feeble bodies cannot handle that amount of magnificence. When we cannot shut off the world on a regular basis, when we try to just be contempt with who we are and never strive for perfection, or try to deal with our own inner struggles alone then we do God and ourselves a great injustice. There is a necessity to set apart time to have a deep conversation with God.

If you are like me it is very difficult to try and sit in silence for a long period of time. When I try to practice *Lectio Divina* the longest I can truly concentrate is roughly 5 min, unless I have some classical music on in the background in which I can last a little longer. But I think as men in the world we are called to a different type of silence. We are called to a silence of hard labor. For example, have you ever noticed when you are doing yard work or cleaning the house in silence there is a much greater opportunity for us to think? When our hands are doing the work our minds are able to relax. I am reminded of one of my favorite paintings by Jefferson David Chalfant simply titled *The Blacksmith*. In that painting there is an old, bearded man that is hammering away at a piece of steel in what looks like his own shop. You can tell that the man is at peace with himself and with the world. His hands are probably as rough as the hammer he is holding and his back as strong as an ox from years of hard labor, but the man has a small grin on his face. The sensation of steel on steel and the peace and quiet that resides between each blow of the hammer keeps this man in his youth and reminds him that he is still full of life and virility. The silence that surrounds him reminds him that he is still a creature of God and that when he is in his place of work he can pray and converse with his Creator, "mano a mano". We can reach this type of prayer with our Lord through the silence of reflection in specific times during our weight lifting and exercise. I truly believe that God made Joseph the foster-father of Jesus because he could teach Jesus about these times of reflection and silence during his hard labor as a carpenter.

> *"God gave us faculties for our use; each of them will receive its proper reward. Then do not let us try to charm them to sleep, but permit them to do their work until divinely called to something higher."*
> – *St. Teresa of Avila* *(italics added)*

I will forever remember when my father and I went on a three-day silent retreat up in the hills of Ohio at the Apostolate for Family Consecration; I have never been so challenged to face myself and to listen for the voice of God. I recall that the first day, during the free time that we had, I decided to go for a run. The entire place was covered in snow and there was absolute silence, not a bird or any other noise to be heard. I can still remember the feeling that it was much too quiet, but then by the third day my mind was at ease and I was able to really listen. It takes quite a bit of practice and determination to allow the noise to stop. "He approaches nearest to the gods who knows how to be silent" was Marcus Porcius Cato's way of saying that the more we are able to create a time to truly listen and stop the chaos that surrounds us, our relationship with the divine will be increased. The old saying, "you have two ears and one mouth, you need to listen twice as much as you talk" is wisdom for the ages. Many of us are too worried about being heard rather than listening. We put such a great deal of importance on our own ideas and ideals that very rarely are we able to just stop and listen. Just as we want to pack on muscle and endurance to our physical bodies in order to be able to stay healthy and tolerate any physical hardships, silence is like a citadel built around our souls, when we keep the noise out so does much of the temptations. We can disregard any of the nonsense that this world offers when we are able to control what we decide to take in. Silence and the ability to listen to our Lord is the engine in which the horsepower of the soul increases. If we desire to increase in holiness then we must desire times of silence as well.

Satan himself fears a man that is able to silence all of the noise because the less we are preoccupied with the things of this world the more we are able to listen to the small hints from God to cultivate a higher sense of our relationship with Him. When Jesus went into the desert for forty days He gave us an excellent example of why we need to have times of silence and that a person craving and achieving these times will upset our greatest enemy. When Moses went up Mount Sinai to listen to God's hallowed voice he went through the struggle of climbing up the mountain before he was able to present himself to the Almighty. I believe that when we are lifting or exercising we have a superb opportunity to have times of silence. I enjoy listening to music when I workout, sometimes orchestras and sometimes a much faster paced music, which is great. But, there is a time right before and right after a person lifts that the world seems to stop. Before you lift there is a feeling of a build up to

In Lorenzo Scupoli's Spiritual Combat he says, "Silence, beloved, is a safe stronghold in the spiritual battle, and a sure pledge of victory. Silence is a friend of him who distrusts self and trusts in God, it is the guardian of prayer and a wonderful help in the attainment of virtue."

something magnificent that is about to happen. You are trying to get yourself in the right mindset to go to war with yourself. All your worries and all the stress of this broken world seem to fall off of your shoulders and you start to only think about one thing, giving the best effort possible. On the other side of the lift, when you are done, there is a time when time seems to stand still and the whole world is at peace. You feel the blood flowing through your muscles and the air going in and out of your lungs. Your mind is in harmony with your body and all seems well. What better times are there to have a conversation with your Savior? What better times are there to stop and listen for God?

Sister Marie-Aimée of Jesus, a Carmelite from Paris, divided the degrees of silence into twelve different categories:

1. *Silence of Speech* which is the most fundamental form of silence.

2. *Bodily Silence* which assists the soul in interior recollection.

3. *Silence of the Senses* which sets a guard over the gateways of our soul.

4. *Silence of the Imagination* which is necessary to bring to silence the unnecessary movements of the emotions, and the meaningless impressions of the fantasy.

5. *Silence of the Memory.* The past must come to silence; otherwise the soul will never come to itself.

6. *Silence from Interior Conversations.* The soul must withdraw itself into the deepest depths of that sanctuary where the inaccessible Majesty of the Holy of Holies dwells.

7. *The Silence of the Heart* which works so that the entire emotive life come to order and find its proper place.

8. *Silence of Self-Love* which is the silence of those who rejoice in their own lowliness.

9. *Silence of the Spirit* which silences the kind of self-seeking which only hinders the working of God.

10. *Silence of Judgment* which refrains not only from sinful harsh judgments of others, but to be reserved in one's own opinions.

11. *Silence of the Will* which silences the anxieties of the heart, the anguish of the soul, to place trust completely in God's loving Providence.

12. *The Silence of Eternity* which is the soul simply resting in God. This is no longer a silence which proceeds from the soul; rather the soul is in silence, because God has enveloped the soul entirely in Himself.

- available at therealpresence.org/chapel

Bodily silence is described as that 'which assists the soul in interior recollection.' Fulton Sheen once said that, "Prayer begins by talking to God, but it ends by listening to Him. In the face of Absolute Truth, silence is the soul's language." Just as I had spoken of before there are specific times when we have the opportunity to take advantage of a time when all is still. Just like the silence before the storm we have a moment of complete serenity, just before and just after we work out. I am a type of person that enjoys getting psyched up, or in other words, getting myself in the right mindset before I lift. I feel that I might be missing something if I don't, plus it is very difficult to hit the weights if you are too relaxed. Just before that time of getting psyched up there is a time that reminds me of what I call a "General Patton" moment (based off of the famous send off speech from the movie *Patton*) when you are looking for those words of exhilaration. This is the time that we need to offer to God, let Him give us that send off speech before we go to war with ourselves. Life doesn't offer enough times as special as those that allow God to be that driving force in our physical lives. Let Him be the General that gives us the speech that makes our blood boil with tenacity. Through the Holy Spirit we are an unconquerable force, we must allow Him time to talk with us and give us the advice and guidance that we need.

'A horrid stillness first invades the ear, And in that silence we the tempest fear.'
— Astroea Redux (1. 7) John Dryden.

The degree of silence that I would like to expound upon is the silence of interior conversation, this one that I struggle with. I have a hard time shutting off my own mind to be able to allow God to speak with and through me. But just as the description details, "the soul must withdraw itself into the deepest depths … where the Holy of Holies dwells" we must commit to a practice of going into our own souls, looking for the heart of our existence which is Jesus Christ Himself, there we can find that inner peace that we all long for, there we can find true silence and a place of reflection. When we reach that deepest part of who we are we must empty any of our ego or pride and allow God to fill that which is empty. "I did never know so full a voice issue from so empty a heart; but the saying is true, 'The empty vessel makes the greatest sound'"—William Shakespeare *The life of King Henry V (Boy at IV, v)*. We must empty our own cup so that God can fill it with the Divine blood. Our souls yearn for it. But how can we empty ourselves if we are never in silence? If we desire to allow God to work within our lives we have got to give Him time to speak to us. This time can be a very sacred and blessed occasion, we can open our ears to that which is almost impossible to hear, we can allow our minds to slow down and let the beauty of God's voice fill our eardrums. Our ears are bombarded with constant noise and distraction; I can't remember the last time I went to sleep without that tiny little ringing in my ear from too much noise during the day.

Once again, our Lord is not one to come right out and say what He wants us to hear. Out of love for us He controls His voice so that we can continue in our voyage to fall deeper and deeper in love with Him. One thing that I have noticed in the Bible is that our Lord either speaks with whispers or He brings down the whole fury of His strength. For example, when Moses was asking the Pharaoh to "Let his people go," through ignorance and pride the Pharaoh did not listen; this was the first whisper of our Lord. Second, through the power of God, Moses turned the sea into a sea of blood; this was a little louder than the first whisper. On and on God continually whispers to Pharaoh what it is that He wants done, until finally the Angel of Death descended upon all of the Egyptians first born sons, this was our Lord at the volume that we mere humans will finally listen. Let us learn from this story to listen to our Lord when He wishes to speak to us. Through our own pride we ignore Him and we go with our own decisions, but in the end ignorance and pride will lead to death.

Another illustration of how often we ignore God's whispers is the fact that there were so many prophecies about Jesus in the Old Testament yet when we had Him here on Earth with us we were completely unaware and we put Him to death.

"Therefore the Lord himself will give you a sign: The virgin will be with child and will give birth to a son, and will call him Immanuel" (Isaiah 7:14).

"The kings of Tarshish and of distant shores will bring tribute to him; the kings of Sheba and Seba will present him gifts" (Psalms 72:10–11).

"Now I am sending my messenger he will prepare the way before me; And the lord whom you seek will come suddenly to his temple; The messenger of the covenant whom you desire — see, he is coming! says the LORD of hosts" (Malachi 3:1).

All of these forewarnings and yet we still put Jesus on the cross. Through our ignorance of the call to holiness and repentance we crucified Love Itself. We must not make the same mistake and through our pride ignore the wisdom of God. We must silence ourselves and allow God to speak to and through us.

Suggested Prayer:

Most divine Master of my soul, I beg you to slow me down. Allow me to listen when you speak and never to grumble or complain when you don't. I long to serve you; help me to reflect upon your love for me when I am able to stop all of the noise of this secular world. In my rare times of true silence I beseech you to come into my unworthy heart.

Amen

X

Thou shalt rack the weights when finished — the one true God is a God of order

Let all things be done decently and in order.

- 1 Corinthians 14:40

The old saying "cleanliness is close to godliness" can be translated to mean "orderliness is close to godliness". In our lives we have so much chaos around us that it is very important to have a sense of order. That order we crave is a gift from God. Without some type of order in our lives we cannot concentrate on that which will bring us closer to our Creator. There are many lessons to be learned through our life in the weight room and one such lesson is finding a sense of order. We naturally desire a sense of organization; we want things to make sense for us. Chaos does not flow well with an All-Knowing and All-Loving Creator and so when we feel a loss of order we have something missing within us. It is the same in the weight room, if we want real progress we cannot think that going to the gym and fooling around, or just going from one piece of equipment to the next is going to allow for any growth. I am a big advocate of making work outs a fun and exciting thing to do but there cannot be disorder within the weight room because this can lead to a lack of improvement or worse, an injury.

Your body builds muscle in some very unique ways. In *High Intensity Training* brought about by Arthur Jones he states that your muscles grow from the largest to the smallest. So, your thigh and gluteus muscles will need to grow before your forearm muscles will. This is very similar with the spiritual life. We must fix our primary faults before we even think about trying to fix our smaller ones. For example, if you have an addiction to pornography, you must strive to fix that problem before you ever attempt to correct any small venial sins you may struggle with. This process will allow you to have an order to correct any problems you have and be able to grow in your spiritual health. This will not be an easy task, many times during our struggles we will fall again and again, but this is what makes us stronger. "No discipline is enjoyable while it is happening — it is painful! But afterward there will be a quiet harvest of right living for those who are trained in this way" (Hebrews 12:11). The same happens when we try to gain muscle and strength.

We can't gain strength in our smaller areas until our larger ones are strong. If a person wanted to build a house, they would not start by building the roof. They would begin by laying the concrete slab and building a solid foundation before they were to start the process of elevation. So it is with our relationship with God, there must be an order of growth so that there can be a solid foundation before we ever decide to start reaching for the heavens. Our foundation is the Catholic Church and the sacraments that it offers us. We cannot accomplish anything divine without the foundation of the most holy Sacraments. In order to build a solid foundation of muscle there is a certain in order in which it must be built as well.

"Civilization begins with order, grows with liberty and dies with chaos" — Will Durant. In this quote from Will Durant the word civilization has a very revealing synonym when put in the context of exercise, and that word is progress. Progress of strength and health is the whole point of lifting weights, if we do not go forward, we go backward. Just as in our spiritual lives there must be progress or else we backslide into old habits or vices, the same goes for our bodies. The progress is dependent upon how well ordered the actions taken have been. Will Durant also states that civilization (progress) grows with liberty. We have a free will to choose what it is that we would like to do; we can either follow God or bow down to the world. We can either find a logical workout routine or we can play around and never progress. Our free choices can either make us the greatest of

"To have his path made clear for him is the aspiration of every human being in our beclouded and tempestuous existence"
— Joseph Conrad.

saints or the worst of demons and that is why progress is dependent upon liberty. Finishing the quote it states that civilization, once again replaced with progress, dies with chaos. Chaos is the state of disorderly conduct and confusion, basically a simple definition of Hell. If we are supposed to further the Kingdom of God in all things then we should never allow chaos into any part of our lives, whether spiritually or physically.

While your body gains muscle in a specific order, your body also needs some things to shock it out of monotonous routines. Just as God created the universe with a certain amount of order and organization, He still allows a random comet or asteroid to fly across the sky and hit another celestial body just to keep things interesting. In order for our muscles to grow we have to 'keep them on their toes' so to speak, we are not meant to drone on with the same old routine, we must consistently throw in a little change. "The art of progress is to preserve order amid change and to preserve change amid order" — Alfred North Whitehead. Our relationship with Christ is very similar. We must keep our prayer lives ordered and our vices in check. But, with our prayer lives it is wise to throw in a new prayer or a new way of speaking with our Lord just so that the relationship continues to grow and envelope your entire life, rather than just one simple area. With our vices, those are counter-acted with virtue. We might have one virtue that is easier to us than the other virtues, say for example, justice, but the vice that we struggle with is jealousy, so, rather than focusing on your ability to be just with your children and neighbors, there is a need to change things a bit and focus on the virtue opposite of the vice you struggle with. Using our example of jealousy we can counteract that vice with humility. So, the order of your life stays the same but the change within it keeps you progressing to a closer relationship with our Lord.

Now, a person cannot speak of Catholic order without talking about the order of the Mass. "... the Mass is exactly the opposite of a Man seeking to be a God. It is a God seeking to be a Man; it is God giving His creative life as such, and restoring the original pattern of their manhood; making not gods, nor beasts, nor angels; but, by the original blast and miracle that makes all things new, turning men into men" — *Magic and Fantasy in Fiction* G. K. Chesterton. The Mass is a continuation of the love story that we have with our Creator. We begin by singing His praises and asking for forgiveness. Then we read about our human history with Him and how much He loves us. Then we cry out to our Savior to continue the sacrifice for our unworthy souls, bread and wine is offered for the sacrifice and God then transforms the gifts we offer into the Body, Blood, Soul, and Divinity of Jesus Christ Himself and allows us to partake. Then, we again sing His praises and thank Him for the continual sacrifice that was celebrated. There must be a specific order to something as mystical and beautiful as the Mass.

The Mass should be such an integral part of our lives that we desire to have that celebration with Him and the thankfulness of what the Mass is that we carry it throughout our day. One way we can resonate the Mass within our own lives is we can use our time of exercise as a guide. We begin by praising God for His kindness and mercy and beg Him to forgive us. We can read a simple quote from scripture and contemplate that during our time in the gym. We can then give up our own bodies as the sacrifice we can offer God and then when we are done we can praise Him for His continual sacrifice He offers to us. I am not putting the time in the gym on the same level as the Mass that would be like comparing a maggot to a pure-bred racehorse. But, what I am suggesting is that we can take the celebration of the Mass with us wherever we go, because Jesus Christ resides within us and that is something that we should celebrate.

With the aim of knowing how we are to order our lives we must look at what it is that we are meant for in this life. Our main mission in this world is to know, love, and serve God. So to be in accordance with the order of our nature this is what we are called to do. "A happy life is one which is in accordance with its own nature"— Seneca. We cannot expect to be happy in this life if our goals are not intended to fulfill that which we are meant for, and we are meant to have a certain amount of order in our lives. As I said before chaos can never lead to a productive life. I know how crazy life can get at times but we must continue to search for that unique balance that order can offer.

"Pray moreover that He may order thy goings that they turn not back unto wickedness, but may go on steadily in the heavenly way of His commandments, and so hasten without any turning aside to the blessed country of the Angels"— St. Anselm.

"The universal order and the personal order are nothing but different expressions and manifestations of a common underlying principle" — Marcus Aurelius, the common underlying principle Aurelius speaks of here is the growing relationship with our Creator through knowing loving, and serving Him. We will never find the balance that we are searching for if our own souls are not in order with what we are called to do. Have you ever noticed how a person that is not living in accordance to the order of our nature will act once he/she has been placed in an inopportune moment? Many times the person will not be able to handle it; they will blame others or will try and drown out the situation with sin upon sin. Many good men that are addicted to pornography can attest to this fact, when caught in use of this devastating addiction they lie, not only to their spouse and themselves but to God, adding the sin of dishonesty to the already deadly sin of lust. Moreover, have you ever noticed how a person that doesn't have their soul in order will not be able to look you in the eye? It is very difficult to look anything face to face when your soul is face to face with darkness. The very order of our nature is designed to be surrounded with the love of God and when we cut off that channel of love we can only deserve and receive fundamental anarchy. "Order is the shape upon which beauty depends"— Pearl S. Buck.

Beyond the humor of the title for this commandment there is a major need to list a couple of common courtesies that should be followed while working out or in a gym. I can remember when I was in college and would work out either at the university weight room or at a local gym and so many times there would be guys that would just be so disrespectful of others and would bring more attention to themselves than a monkey in a zoo. So, because of that I felt the need to list some things that we can do in order to be good Christians in the gym. "Order is Heaven's first law"— Alexander Pope.

Do not talk to others while they are lifting

→ Address others in between sets, but a conversation can wait until after the work out

Show up expecting to lift

→ Fooling around or people watching is not why you go to a gym

Clean up after yourself

→ Rack the weights

→ Use a towel on yourself and the equipment after a lift

Dress appropriately

→ You are a child of God, not a piece of meat to be gawked at

Be positive and constructive

→ Never be negative to others, you are all there to improve

Ask for a spot and offer to give one

→ If you are going heavy, ask politely for a spot, not only for safety but also to keep yourself from making a scene

→ If anyone asks for a spot don't be too cool to help

Don't hog any equipment

→ Part of the beauty of High Intensity Training is that you are never at the same machine or bench for very long

Don't douse yourself with cologne before you workout

→ Nothing is worse than breathing heavily and having to take in those hemicals

A little grunting is ok, but don't try to be Tarzan in the gym

→ You shouldn't draw a lot of attention to yourself

→ If you are in a home gym with some buddies, then some cave-man grunts are ok

And last but definitely not least:

LEAVE YOUR EGO AT HOME!

As in the Olympic Games it is not the most beautiful and strongest who receive the crown, but those who actually enter the combat. For from those come the victors, so it is those who act that win rightly what is noble and good in life.

Aristotle, Nichomachean Ethics

Example Workout Routines

"Out of intense complexities intense simplicities emerge."

- Winston Churchill

Before I give a few examples of workout routines that have worked for me in the past and have been proven to work I would like to speak about a certain type of workout that I have prescribed to. It is called High Intensity Training or HIT for short. This type of training was brought about in the 1970's by a man named Arthur Jones, founder of Nautilus. The training is focused on quality repetitions, usually only one set to the point of momentary muscular failure. The fundamental principles are that exercise should be brief, infrequent, and intense, also focusing on recovery. One of the best examples of the power of these workouts is the alpha-male in a lion's den, he is always the largest, most muscular and most powerful of the lions. The alpha male does not do any of the hunting and sleeps almost all day, but, when it comes time to protect his lionesses and cubs his actions are quick and amazingly intense. I believe that HIT works extremely well for people that have regular lives and cannot workout for hours on end. Most of the workouts only last around 20–30 min at most. Some of the most famous bodybuilders have subscribed to HIT including, Casey Viator, Mike and Ray Mentzer, Sergio Oliva, Lee Labrada and one of my favorites, Dorian Yates. Original HIT principles started by Arthur Jones are also highly against any steroid use or any drugs to speak of. The diets are only concerned with eating a healthy, balanced diet and not overloading on protein or under eating carbohydrates. HIT is highly logical and has been proven through results. I am a big fan of changing your routines on a regular basis. Every 3–4 weeks your muscles start becoming used to the effort that is put on them when you work out on a regular basis, therefore a changeup is needed. Also, droning on with the same routine over and over again takes all of the fun out of weight lifting. Remember, ALWAYS use proper form and never use more weight than is reasonable, an injury can only set you back. "Hence diversity and change are to be accounted for immediately by motion + matter; while ultimately the sole efficient cause of all things is nothing else than the Will of God" — St. Bernard of Clairveux.

Example #1:

This workout is to be performed 2–3 times a week. I have actually done this workout one time a week in order to concentrate on recovery as well. Aim to keep the repetitions between 6–8 reps; if the reps go higher increase the weight on the next workout. The repetitions should be performed at a steady speed, 2–4 seconds on the negative action and 2–4 seconds on the positive action. On average, with only short brakes between sets, you can finish this workout in 20–25 minutes.

- Barbell Squats: 1 set 6–8 reps

- Deadlift: 1 set 6–8 reps

- Bench press: 1 set 6–8 reps

- Pull-ups: 1 set to failure, try to throw in some negatives (concentrate on the lowering of your body slowly but surely, try and take 10-15 seconds to lower your body, you'll be amazed at the results)

- Shoulder Overhead Press: 1 set 6–8 reps

- Barbell curls: 1 set 6–8 reps

- Triceps dumbbell extensions: 1 set (each arm) 6–8 reps

- Barbell Shrugs: 1 set –8 reps

- Weighted Calf raises: 1 set (each calf) 8–10 reps

- Wrist Curls with a crooked bar: 1 set to failure

- Abdominal Crunches: 1 set to failure

- Abdominal Leg Raises (Lying or Hanging): 1 set to failure

Example #2:

This workout breaks the muscles down into groups. Still allow the 2–4 seconds on the negative and positive actions. We now throw in some secondary movements to hit different areas of the muscle. These workouts are to be performed within about an 8 day period, less or more depending on how well you are recovering. I suggest very little rest between sets. These workouts do not take much time at all.

Day 1:

- Chest and Biceps

- Bench (Incline, Decline, or Flat) Press: 1 set 6–8 reps

- Dumbbell Flyes (Incline or Flat): 1 set 8–10 reps

- Barbell Curls: 1 set 6–8 reps

- Dumbbell Hammer Curls: 1 set (per arm) 8–10 reps

- Abdominal crunches: 1 set to failure

Day 2:

- Back and Triceps

- Deadlift: 1 set 6–8 reps

- Bent-over Barbell Rows: 1 set 8–10 reps

- Pull-ups: 1 set to failure, try to throw in some negatives

- Skull Crushers: 1 set 6–8 reps

- Dumbbell Triceps Extension: 1 set 8–10

Day 3:

- Legs and Shoulders

- Barbell Squat: 1 set 6–8 reps

- Leg Extensions: 1 set till failure (try and pause at the top of the movement)

- Leg Curls: 1 set till failure

- Weighted Calf raises: 1 set (each calf) till failure

- Overhead Shoulder Press: 1 set 6–8 reps

- Bent Arm Dumbbell Lateral Raises: 1 set 8–10 reps

- Barbell Shrugs: 1 set 8–10 reps

- Abdominal Leg raises: 1 set to failure

- Oblique Abdominal Side Bends (Weighted): 1 set to failure

Example #3:

This is a 2-day split routine. I would suggest that you only do this routine once or twice a week. If you would like perform the routine more often you can wait 48 hours before starting over. Because there are many very effective abdominal workouts choose one or two that you enjoy and put them on both days.

Day 1:

- Barbell Squat: 1 set 6–8 reps

- Deadlift: 1 set 6–8 reps

- Bench Press: 1 set 6–8 reps

- Bent Arm Dumbbell Lateral Raises: 1 set 8–10 reps

- Barbell Curls: 1 set 6–8 reps

- Close grip bench press: 1 set 6–8 reps

Day 2:

- Leg Extensions: 1 set to failure

- Leg Curls: 1 set to failure

- Decline (or Incline) Bench Press: 1 set 6–8 reps

- Pull-ups: 1 set to failure

- Or Bent over Barbell Rows: 1 set 6–8 reps

- Shoulder Overhead Press: 1 set 6–8 reps

- Hammer curls: 1 set 6–8 reps

- Triceps extension: 1 set (each arm) 6–8 reps

- Weighted Calf Raises: 1 set (each leg) to failure

There are many different lifts that can be substituted for any one of these exercise routines. I am a fan of compound exercise, or those that use many different muscles at once, so I recommend keeping those in your routines.

Cardio Recommendations: Depending on your goals I suggest cardio 2–3 times a week. See *Fit for Eternal Life* by Dr. Kevin Vost for the different types of cardio practices.

Ode of a Catholic Bodybuilder

My body is a temple,

Ready for war,

I train to stay healthy,

To better serve the Lord.

My King desires perfection,

In mind, body and soul,

Through blood, sweat and tears

My body will pay the toll.

Strength and Honor,

Discipline and Prayer,

Unworthy of heaven,

But my King wishes me there.

I will prepare my body,

Educate my mind,

Through my loving Queen,

My soul will thrive.

My power will increase,

My muscles will grow,

Years of enemy temptation,

But I will serve God alone.

Book Recommendations

Books by Dr. Kevin Vost Psy.D.

- Fit for Eternal Life

- Memorize the Faith! (and Most Anything Else): Using the Methods of the Great Catholic Medieval Memory Masters

- From Atheism to Catholicism: How Scientists and Philosophers Led Me to Truth

- St. Albert the Great: Champion of Faith and Reason

- Unearthing Your Ten Talents

- Three Irish Saints: A Study in Spiritual Styles

- Memorize the Reasons!

The Rosary Workout by Peggy Bowes

Tending the Temple

- by Dr. Kevin Vost Psy.D., Peggy Bowes and Shane Kapler

The Catholic Workout by Michael Carrera

The Catholic Ideal: Exercise and Sports by Robert Feeney

Books by Fr. Joe Classen

- Hunting for God, Fishing for the Lord

- Meat and Potatoes Catholicism

- Tracking Virtue, Conquering Vice

- The Essentials of Catholic Spirituality

Spiritual Combat by Lorenzo Scupoli

***Theology of The Body* for Beginners by Christopher West**

Man and Woman He Created Them: A *Theology of The Body* — John Paul II

CPSIA information can be obtained at www.ICGtesting.com
Printed in the USA
LVOW131013200612

286904LV00003B/144/P

9 780984 486496